W0091499

Beta-Blockers in Heart Failure

John JV McMurray BSc MD FRCP FESC FACC

Professor of Medical Cardiology
Clinical Research Initiative
in Heart Failure, University of Glasgow
and Honorary Consultant Cardiologist
Western Infirmary
Glasgow
UK

Martin J Kendall MD FRCP

Professor of Clinical Pharmacology
Department of Medicine
Queen Elizabeth Hospital
Birmingham
UK

MARTIN DUNITZ

© Martin Dunitz Ltd 2002

First published in the United Kingdom in 2002 by Martin Dunitz Ltd
The Livery House, 7–9 Pratt Street, London NW1 0AE

Tel: +44-(0)20-7482-2202
Fax: +44-(0)20-7267-0159
E-mail: info.dunitz@tandf.co.uk
Website: http://www.dunitz.co.uk

Although every effort has been made to ensure that drug doses and other
information are presented accurately in this publication, the ultimate
responsibility rests with the prescribing physician. Neither the publishers
nor the authors can be held responsible for errors for any consequences
arising from the use of information contained herein. For detailed prescribing
information or instructions on the use of any product or procedure discussed
herein, please consult the prescribing information or instructional material
issued by the manufacturer.

A CIP catalogue record for this book is available from the British Library

ISBN 1-85317-902-7

Distributed in the USA by
Fulfilment Center
Taylor & Francis
7625 Empire Drive
Florence, KY 41042, USA
Toll Free Tel: 1-800-634-7064
Email: cserve@routledge_ny.com

Distributed in Canada by
Taylor & Francis
74 Rolark Drive
Scarborough
Ontario M1R G2, Canada
Toll Free Tel: 1-877-226-2237
Email: tal_fran@istar.ca

Distributed in the rest of the world by
ITPS Limited
Cheriton House
North Way, Andover
Hampshire SP10 5BE, UK
Tel: +44 (0) 1264 332424
Email: reception@itps.co.uk

Printed and bound in Italy by Printer Trento S.r.l.

Contents

Beta blockers and heart failure – a historical perspective

Beta-blockers were first used to treat hypertension and angina after reports on their efficacy by Pritchard and colleagues in 1964.[1] In the early days propranolol was the only drug in clinical use. It soon became evident that this drug was more effective and better tolerated than other antihypertensive drugs available at that time, but that it could cause a serious deterioration if given to patients with asthma or heart failure. It therefore became accepted that both asthma and heart failure were absolute contraindications to the use of beta-blockers. Asthma remains an absolute contraindication. However, over the period 1994–1999 beta-blockers changed from being contraindicated in patients with heart failure to being judged potentially the most effective form of treatment for this serious disorder.

Workers at the Hammersmith Hospital in London started to think that beta-blockers might have a beneficial effect in some forms of heart failure in 1964, the year of the first publication on propranolol in hypertension.[1] They were studying hypertrophic obstructive cardiomyopathy and recognized the need to reduce outflow tract obstruction and reduce the raised left ventricular diastolic pressure.[2] The paradoxical effects of catecholamines on diastolic pressure were known at that time, and Cohen and Braunwald[3] were the first to study the effects of beta-blockers on left ventricular diastolic pressure. Subsequently, the adverse effects of exercise producing tachycardia and a reduction in stroke volume in hypertrophic obstructive cardiomyopathy were treated by beta-blockade by Edwards and colleagues in 1970,[4] also at the Hammersmith Hospital.

In the mid-1970s, Finn Waagstein and colleagues in Gothenburg, Sweden, recognized the importance of slowing heart rate in patients with heart failure and considered the possibility that beta-blockade might be a suitable long-term treatment for chronic heart failure.[5,6] They had the courage to believe in their haemodynamic assessments despite the almost universal belief that beta-blockade would be fatal in patients with severe heart failure. They also recognized the need to stabilize the patient on optimal therapy, to start with very low doses, to monitor very closely, and to anticipate that it might take several weeks or months to achieve the full benefits of beta-blockade.

The early studies in Gothenburg were rejected and ignored by the cardiological community. It was difficult to persuade editors to publish the data and difficult to obtain funding for major studies. However, over the next 10 years beta-blockers were used extensively to treat hypertension and angina. They were also shown to have a substantial effect on total mortality and sudden death in patients who had had an acute myocardial infarction.[7–10] Not surprisingly many of the post-MI patients had heart failure and these patients were also helped by beta-blockade.[8,10] These results, and the increasing number of small studies that showed beneficial effects of beta-blockade in heart failure, argued strongly for setting up a placebo-controlled trial of beta-blocker therapy in heart failure even though many still regarded such a trial as unethical and doomed to failure.

In 1993, the metoprolol dilated cardiomyopathy trial was published.[11] In that study, patients with severe heart failure were carefully titrated from very small doses of metoprolol up to standard doses, and the effects on mortality and need for transplantation were compared with placebo. Although metoprolol had an impact on the combined end-point of mortality plus transplantation, some critics judged this a negative trial because mortality was not reduced significantly. Fortunately, the results of this and many other studies provided sufficient evidence to persuade the clinical investigators and pharmaceutical companies to work together to set up the major clinical trials of beta-blockers in heart failure, which are described in this book.

Heart failure

The consensus recommendations for the management of chronic heart failure published in the *American Journal of Cardiology* in 1999[12] define heart failure as a complex clinical syndrome that can result from any cardiac disorder that impairs the ability of the ventricles to eject blood.

Key factors of this disorder are that:

- It is a common medical condition and is becoming more common
- It usually causes dyspnoea and fatigue, which reduce exercise tolerance and fluid retention, leading to pulmonary and peripheral oedema
- There are many different causes but coronary artery disease is the most common and may lead to left ventricular dysfunction in two thirds of patients.
- It is usually progressive
- It has a poor prognosis
- Death may be sudden or result from progression of the heart failure.

Heart failure afflicts about 4.8 million people in the USA, with 400,000–700,000 new cases each year.[13–15] In the UK, heart failure accounts for 5% of all admissions to hospital medical beds and has a prevalence of 3–20 per 1000 population, though the incidence is much higher in those over 65 years of age.[16]

In recent years, interest in the treatment of heart failure has increased enormously. There are many reasons for this but probably the most important is the fact that for the first time a group of drugs, the angiotensin converting enzyme (ACE) inhibitors, were shown to have a beneficial effect on the life expectancy of patients with heart failure. The Cooperative North Scandinavian Enalapril Survival Study (CONSENSUS) was a landmark study and showed that enalapril could reduce all-cause mortality by 27% in a group of patients with severe heart failure.[17] The 1-year mortality in the placebo group was 52%. Interestingly, the entire reduction in mortality was in deaths from progressive heart failure. There was no difference between groups in the incidence of sudden cardiac death. Many other studies have confirmed the beneficial effects of ACE inhibitors in heart failure[18] and in post-MI patients.[19] These trials transformed the management of heart failure such that by the mid-1990s most patients with heart failure were being treated with diuretics and an ACE inhibitor. Some were also on digoxin.

ACE inhibitors have improved the outlook of patients with heart failure but they still have a poor prognosis. Precise figures depend on the population of patients studied and are influenced by many factors, particularly the severity of the heart failure and the age of the patients. In Table 1 the number of deaths in the placebo groups of the four trials to be described in this book[20–22] are presented together with a rough estimate of the annual mortality.

Perhaps more useful are the data from MERIT-HF — the largest study — which shows that in the placebo groups the mortality rates were 7.1%, 13.2% and 24.9% per patient

Table 1
Mortality rates in placebo groups of major beta-blocker heart failure studies.

	US Carvedilol	CIBIS-II	MERIT-HF	COPERNICUS
Number in group	398	1320	2001	1133
Duration of study (months)	6.5	15	12	11
Number of deaths	31	228	217	190
Estimated mortality in 1 year (%)	14.3	13.8	10.8	18.5

year of follow-up for NYHA Class II, III and IV patients respectively.[22] Thus, optimal treatment including ACE inhibitors but not beta-blockers is still associated with a high mortality. Most cancers have a better prognosis than heart failure and very few are as lethal as NYHA Class IV heart failure.

Heart failure is also a major cause of morbidity and many of the patients require frequent admissions to hospital. Recognizing the importance of this, the investigators in the major trials have collected and presented the data not only on mortality but also on hospital admissions. In MERIT-HF[23] 767 (38%) of 2001 patients in the placebo group died or were admitted to hospital (for any reason). In the placebo group of CIBIS-II[21] 463 (35%) of 1320 patients had a cardiovascular death or were admitted to hospital for a cardiovascular disorder.

A treatment for heart failure should:

1. Improve symptoms, ie reduce fatigue, dyspnoea and oedema and improve exercise tolerance
2. Slow the prognosis of the underlying disease
3. Improve cardiac function.

4. Reduce the high mortality rates from sudden death and progressive heart failure
5. Reduce the number and duration of hospital admissions for heart failure.

The four major studies described in this book were designed to determine how effectively the three beta-blockers carvedilol, bisoprolol and metoprolol achieve these aims.

References

1. Pritchard BRC, Gillam PMS. Use of propranolol in treatment of hypertension. *BMJ* 1964; **2:** 725.
2. Cohen J, Effat H, Goodwin JF, Oakley CM, Steiner RE. Hypertrophic obstructive cardiomyopathy. *Br Heart J* 1964; **26:** 16.
3. Cohen LS, Braunwald E. Amelioration of angina pectoris in idiopathic hypertrophic subaortic stenosis with beta-adrenergic blockade. *Circulation* 1967; **35:** 847.
4. Edwards RHT, Kristinsson A, Warrell DA, Goodwin JF. Effects of propranolol on response to exercise in hypertrophic obstructive cardiomyopathy. *Br Heart J* 1970; **32:** 219.
5. Waagstein F, Caidahl K, Wallentin I, Bergh CH, Hjalmarson A. Long term beta-blockade in dilated cardiomyopathy: effects of short and long-term metoprolol treatment followed by withdrawal and readministration of metoprolol. *Circulation* 1989; **90:** 551–63.
6. Waagstein F, Hjalmarson A, Varnauskas E, Wallentin I. Effect of chronic beta-adrenergic receptor blockade in congestive cardiomyopathy. *Br Heart J* 1975; **37:** 1022.
7. The Norwegian Multicenter Study Group. Timolol-induced reduction in mortality and reinfarction in patients surviving acute myocardial infarction. *N Engl J Med* 1981; **304:** 801–7.
8. Beta Blocker Heart Attack Research Group. A randomized trial of propranolol in patients with acute myocardial infarction. 1. Mortality results. *JAMA* 1982; **247:** 1707–13.
9. Olsson G, Wikstrand J, Warnold I, et al. Metoprolol-induced reduction in postinfarction mortality: pooled results from five double-blind randomized trials. *Eur Heart J* 1992; **13:** 28–32.
10. Herlitz J, Waagstein F, Lindqvist J, Swedberg K. Effect of metoprolol on the prognosis for patients with suspected acute myocardial infarction and indirect signs of congestive heart failure (A subgroup analysis of the Göteborg metoprolol trial). *Am J Cardiol* 1997; **80**(9B): 40J–44J.

11. Waagstein F, Bristow M, Swedberg K, et al, of the Metoprolol Dilated Cardiomyopathy (MDC) Trial Study Group. Beneficial effects of metoprolol in idiopathic dilated cardiomyopathy. *Lancet* 1993; **342:** 1441–6.

12. Packer M, Cohn JN. Consensus Recommendations for the management of chronic heart failure. *Am J Cardiol* 1999; **83**(2A): 1A–3A.

13. American Heart Association. Heart and stroke statistical update. Dallas: AHA, 1998.

14. Massie BM, Shah NB. Evolving trends in the epidemiologic factors of heart failure: rationale for preventive strategies and comprehensive disease management. *Am Heart J* 1997; **133:** 703–12.

15. O'Connell JB, Bristow MR. Economic impact of heart failure in the United States: time for a different approach. *J Heart Lung Transplant* 1994; **13:** S107–S112.

16. Davis RC, Hobbs FDR, Lip GYH. ABC of heart failure. History and epidemiology. *BMJ* 2000; **320:** 39–42.

17. The Consensus Trial Group. Effect of enalapril on mortality in severe congestive heart failure: results of the Cooperative North Scandinavian Enalapril Survival Study (CONSENSUS). *N Engl J Med* 1987; **316:** 1429–35.

18. Cleland JGF. The clinical course of heart failure and its modification by ACE inhibitors: insights from recent clinical trials. *Eur Heart J* 1995; **15:** 125–30.

19. Torp-Pedersen C, Kober L, TRACE Study Group. Effect of ACE inhibitor trandolapril on life expectancy of patients with reduced left-ventricular function after acute myocardial infarction. *Lancet* 1999; **354:** 9–12.

20. Packer M, Bristow MR, Cohn et al, and the US Carvedilol Heart Failure Study Group. The effect of carvedilol on morbidity and mortality in patients with chronic heart failure. *N Engl J Med* 1996; **334:** 1349–55.

21. CIBIS-II Investigators and Committees. The cardiac insufficiency bisoprolol study II (CIBIS-II): a randomised trial. *Lancet* 1999; **353:** 9–13.

22. MERIT-HF Study Group. Effect of metoprolol CR/XL in chronic heart failure: metoprolol CR/XL randomised intervention trial in congestive heart failure (MERIT-HF). *Lancet* 1999; **353:** 2001–7

23. Hjalmarson A, Goldstein S, Fagerberg B, et al. Effects of controlled-release metoprolol on total mortality, hospitalizations, and well-being in patients with heart failure: the Metoprolol CR/XL Randomized Intervention Trial in congestive heart failure (MERIT-HF). MERIT-HF Study Group. *JAMA* 2000; **283:** 1295–302.

Mode of action of beta-blockers

Introduction

Beta-blockers have been used for many years to treat patients with hypertension and angina and those who are having or have recovered from a myocardial infarction. They lower blood pressure and reduce the frequency and severity of attacks of chest pain in angina. More importantly in all these patients they reduce cardiovascular complications, particularly myocardial infarction, re-infarctions and sudden death.[1-3]

For patients with heart failure, the aims of treatment have been defined in the first chapter. Beta-blockers achieve these aims by their effects on a number of processes, many of which are interlinked.

In this chapter we will consider:

- The benefit that may result from counteracting the effects of catecholamine excess
- Data on the effect of beta-blockers on coronary artery disease, derived from:
  1. Laboratory data
  2. Clinical trials.

The role of the autonomic nervous system

The major consequences of myocardial injury or disease are a reduction in cardiac output and a fall in blood pressure. The body responds to any fall in blood pressure and the consequent reduction in tissue perfusion by increasing cardiac output, increasing peripheral resistance, and by promoting salt and water retention. These effects are largely achieved by stimulation of the sympathetic nervous system and the renin angiotensin system.

Increased sympathetic activity:

- Increases heart rate and cardiac output mainly via the beta$_1$ receptors
- Increases peripheral resistance via alpha-mediated vasoconstriction
- Increases renin release, raising plasma concentration of angiotensin II and aldosterone, which produces further vasoconstriction and promotes salt and water retention.

This would be an ideal response in a young person with a normal heart who has a severe haemorrhage. In an older person with a diseased heart this series of responses is potentially damaging.

In heart failure, plasma adrenaline and noradrenaline are markedly raised. Furthermore, the more severe the heart failure the higher the plasma concentrations,[4–6] and the higher the plasma noradrenaline the worse the prognosis.[7] The raised catecholamines have many adverse effects that may be counteracted by beta-blockers. These will be considered under four headings:

1. Haemodynamic
2. Electrical mechanisms
3. Cellular mechanism
4. Oxidative stress.

Haemodynamic

Sympathetic over-activity or catecholamine excess will increase heart rate, reduce heart rate variability and have other effects on cardiac function.

Heart rate

A high resting heart rate has been associated with a poor prognosis in several clinical studies (Table 2). Several epidemiological studies have shown an association between resting heart rate and death from cardiovascular disease and from other causes.[8–12] Heart rate is also an important prognostic index of cardiovascular risk in patients before, during and after a coronary event.[9,13,14] Hjalmarsson and colleagues,[13] for example, have shown that after an infarct those with a resting heart rate over 90 beats per minute have a 2.7 times greater risk of dying than those with a heart rate of 60 beats per minute or less. Further, the increase in heart rate that occurs in the early hours of the day is associated with an increased incidence of cardio-

Table 2

Populations in whom a relation between heart rate and prognosis has been shown

No.	Study population	Endpoint	Reference
1	Epidemiological studies	Coronary artery disease	Dyer, 1980[8] Gillum, 1988[10] Gillum, 1991[11]
2	Patients with ischaemic heart disease	Cardiovascular mortality	Kannel, 1987[9] Shaper, 1993[12]
3	Hypertensive men	Total mortality	Gillman, 1993[111]
4	Acute myocardial infarction	Total mortality	Gunderson, 1986[112] Kjekshus, 1986[21] Hjalmarson, 1990[13] ISIS-2 Study Group[15]
5	Heart failure	Sudden death	Kjekshus, 1999[19] Moser, 1994[14]

vascular events, particularly sudden death[14] and new infarcts.[15]

There are many adverse consequences of persistent tachycardia. An increase in heart rate increases heart work and therefore oxygen demand. Furthermore, the associated shortening of diastole reduces left ventricular filling time and reduces the time during which blood can flow from the epicardial coronary arteries through the perforating vessels to the endocardium. Also, the short periods of flow are associated with increased sheer stress, other mechanical stresses and enhanced platelet aggregation.[16,17] The importance of heart rate in relation to myocardial blood supply is well illustrated by the effect of tachycardia on infarct development. In dogs subjected to acute coronary occlusions, a reduction in heart rate from 150 to 75 beats per minute profoundly improves myocardial metabolism and reduces the area of ischaemia.[18] Studies in man have shown that during infarction, lowering the heart rate decreases the rate of infarct development as measured by creatine kinase release, and may reduce the size of the infarct.[19–21]

Tachycardia is a prominent feature of heart failure, associated with raised plasma noradrenaline concentrations, which can be used as a marker of left ventricular dysfunction[6] and a predictor of survival.[7] In a subgroup study of the SAVE trial, St John Sutton and colleagues[22] noted that in patients with left ventricular dysfunction, heart rate was an important predictor of cardiovascular death. Similarly in the CONSENSUS trial[23] those with baseline heart rates above 85 beats per minute, particularly those in the placebo group, had the worst prognosis. Also, in a study of amiodarone in heart failure, a subgroup with heart rates above 90 beats per minute benefited from the drug's heart rate slowing effect with a 38% reduction in mortality, mostly due to a decrease in sudden deaths.[24]

The serious adverse consequences of an increased heart rate and the need to correct this provide one good reason for using a beta-blocker to treat heart failure. It is important to choose a beta-blocker that will reduce heart rate and to prescribe a dose large enough to achieve a marked reduction in heart rate. It is of interest that the effect of bisoprolol in the first CIBIS Study[25] (maximum dose 5.0 mg) was less than in CIBIS-II[26] (maximum dose 10.0 mg), as discussed later. Further beta-blockers with intrinsic sympathomimetic activity (ISA), which tend not to produce bradycardia, have had little effect in post-infarct patients.[1,21] Although it has been suggested that bucindolol, the beta-blocker used in the BEST trial,[27] appeared to have less effect than bisoprolol in CIBIS-II[26] or metoprolol in MERIT-HF[28] because it had ISA, this is now thought not to be the explanation.

Kjekshus and Gullestad,[19] in their review of heart rate as a therapeutic target in heart failure, have shown a direct correlation between reduction in heart rate and reduction in mortality. This critically important observation was based on results from 14 studies. Further information to support the relation between heart rate and survival will be obtained from more detailed analysis of the large trials. However, an analysis of the prognostic value of changes in haemodynamic variables obtained in the first CIBIS study[25] has shown convincingly that change in heart rate over time had the highest predictive value for survival.[29]

Heart-rate variability (HRV)
Heart-rate changes in normal resting individuals are a response to haemodynamic changes during respiration and are mediated by the autonomic nervous system. Analysis of HRV can provide non-invasive assessment of a patient's autonomic function. In heart failure the reduction in overall variability is attributed to an autonomic imbalance caused by increased sympathetic and decreased vagal activity.[30,31] In post-MI patients, decreased HRV is associated with a poor prognosis.[32] There is evidence to suggest

that beta-blockers may improve the autonomic imbalance that leads to reduced HRV, not only by reducing sympathetic tone but also by increasing vagal tone.[33–36]

A detailed analysis of the subgroup of patients in the first CIBIS study[29] showed that bisoprolol increased HRV or beat-to-beat variability, but only in those with the largest R-R interval. This can be interpreted as showing that in treatment of heart failure, when beta-blockers effectively slow heart rate, they can correct the autonomic imbalance that is associated with a poor prognosis. Increases in vagal tone may therefore contribute to the beneficial effects of beta-blockers in heart failure.

Other haemodynamic effects

Although many of the haemodynamic benefits of beta-blockade in heart failure may be attributable directly or indirectly to the reduction in heart rate, there is some evidence that beta-blockers have additional effects. In a study by Andersson and colleagues[37] a subgroup of patients with cardiomyopathy were put on metoprolol and then subjected to atrial pacing. The authors commented that "when myocardial recovery has been achieved by metoprolol, the improved cardiac function is not adversely affected by higher heart rate." They attributed this to an improved force-frequency relation.

In short, there is evidence that beta-blockers:

- Increase ejection fraction[38]
- Reduce end-systolic volume[39]
- Improve ventricular incoordination[40]
- Improve ventricular filling time[41]
- Help to prevent the remodelling process.[42–44]

In a meta-analysis of 18 double blind, placebo controlled trials involving 3023 patients with heart failure, the mean left ventricular ejection fraction (LVEF) was 23 ± 4% in the placebo group and 31 ± 4% in the beta-blocker group — a very highly significant increase of 29% on beta-blockers. This increase is much greater than has been shown by any other therapeutic agent, and 3–5 times greater than that shown by ACE-inhibitors.[38]

Electrical mechanisms

Since at least half of those with heart failure die suddenly, the potential to reduce the risk of sudden death is an important attribute of beta-blockers. Catecholamines increase abnormal automaticity, triggered activity and re-entry in diseased myocardium.[45] Key clinical studies, described later, have shown convincingly that beta-blockers do reduce the risk of sudden death. Although further studies of the mechanisms involved are needed, the benefits have been largely attributed to the capacity of beta-blockers to counteract the arrhythmogenic effects of catecholamines and also slow heart rate. An effect on vagal tone,[33–36] mediated via the autonomic centres in the brain, may also be important.

Three interesting animal studies show the efficacy of beta-blockers as a means of reducing the risk of death from ventricular fibrillation (VF) in animals subjected to acute myocardial ischaemia. Parker and colleagues in Houston[46] used a pig model, having shown that an acute coronary occlusion followed by psychosocial stress provoked VF in a large proportion of the animals. They then showed that a small dose of propranolol introduced into the cerebral ventricles significantly reduced the incidence of VF.

Delsperger and colleagues in Iowa[47] used a dog model in which renal hypertension induced left ventricular hypertrophy. They then produced acute myocardial ischaemia, which frequently caused VF. Pre-treatment with enalapril or metoprolol reduced the left ventricular hypertrophy, but although metoprolol reduced the risk of VF, enalapril did not.

Ablad and colleagues in Gothenburg[48] used a rabbit model pretreated with placebo, atenolol or metoprolol and then subjected to acute coronary occlusion. Interestingly metoprolol reduced the risk of VF whereas atenolol did not. The authors attributed this difference to the fact that the lipophilic metoprolol was better able to reach the autonomic centre in the brain.

Cellular mechanisms

It has been known for many years that catecholamines are toxic to heart muscle[44,49–51] and that focal myocarditis has been described in patients with a phaeochromocytoma. These adverse effects have been attributed to:

- Depletion of high energy phosphates[44]
- Alterations in calcium handling at the level of the sarcoplasmic reticulum[52]
- Metabolic substrate utilization[52]
- Cytokine expression[43]
- Accelerated apoptosis.[51,53,54]

Some of these can be considered together as a disturbance in myocardial energetics.[55] This syndrome may be characterised by limited aerobic function and limited ATP-ase production by mitochondria that leads to a state of energy depletion.[52,55,56] Treatment with metoprolol improves left ventricular dysfunction[56,57] and improves the myocardial efficiency of the failing heart.[58] Another contributory factor in the development of metabolic dysfunction in heart failure is catecholamine-induced lipolysis. Free fatty acids are a less efficient energy source for the myocardium and lead to ATP-ase wastage. Beta-blockade using metoprolol corrects the hypermetabolic state by increasing dependency on carbohydrate and away from free fatty acid oxidation.[58]

Oxidative stress

One of the toxic effects of catecholamine excess is the production of free radicals and damage resulting from oxidative stress.[59] In heart failure, circulating free radicals may contribute to disease progression and perhaps promote apoptosis. By measuring markers of free radical damage or antioxidant capacity, several studies have shown that patients with heart failure are at risk from free radical damage.[60–63] Ferrari and colleagues[63] have produced an interesting review of the potential role of oxidative stress in ischaemic heart disease. This subject has received considerable attention because carvedilol has antioxidant properties.[64–66] However, a more recent study suggests that metoprolol may be equally effective as an antioxidant.[59] The clinical relevance of oxidative stress and the potential role for antioxidants in the management of heart failure is uncertain. It is possible that one of the effects (probably one of the less important effects) of beta-blockers is to act as an antioxidant.

Beta-blockers and coronary artery disease – laboratory data

Beta-blockers may also have a beneficial impact on the underlying disorder, which in most patients with heart failure is coronary artery disease. Since high blood pressure, tachycardia and a stressed personality predispose to coronary disease, and atheromatous lesions tend to occur at sites of wall stress and high turbulence, beta-blockers might be expected to reduce atheroma formation. Animal data provide evidence that they do. Thubrikar and colleagues[67] studied atheroma formation in rabbit aortas and showed that beta-blockers reduce lipoprotein uptake. Of considerable interest is the work of Kaplan and colleagues, who studied stress in monkeys by moving dominant animals from group to group. These animals had to keep establishing their dominance, a stressful process that resulted in endothelial damage — the first step towards atheroma formation.

In separate studies, both propranolol and metoprolol pre-treatment prevented endothelial damage.[68–70] Propranolol has also been shown to prevent atheroma in rabbits fed a diet high in cholesterol.[71]

Though there is evidence that most antihypertensives can reduce atheroma formation in an animal model, the data on beta-blockers are particularly persuasive.[69] In addition to their haemodynamic actions beta-blockers may also reduce lipid binding to endothelium and arterial wall proteoglycans.[72] There is also evidence that beta-blockers may reduce platelet aggregation,[73,74] and increase prostacyclin formation.[75] More excitingly a low dose of metoprolol CR/XL (25mg once daily) has been shown to reduce the rate of progression of intima media thickness in the carotid arteries of symptomless patients with atheromatous plaques.[76] This suggests that metoprolol may have a favourable effect on atherosclerosis development.[76]

Beta-blockers and coronary artery disease – clinical data

Hypertension

Hypertension is one of the major risk factors for coronary artery disease and the major risk factor for cerebrovascular disease (stroke). The key aim in treating hypertension is, therefore, to prevent these complications. All forms of effective antihypertensive therapy will reduce the risk of stroke, particularly in elderly hypertensive patients.[77–80] Data showing the efficacy of antihypertensive drugs in preventing coronary events, particularly sudden death, were less consistent and less persuasive. However, STOP-Hypertension[78] showed that beta-blockers or diuretics do reduce the risk of coronary events in the elderly. STOP 2[81] showed that in the elderly a calcium channel blocker or an ACE inhibitor was as effective as a beta-blocker or diuretic regimen.

The potential role of beta-blockers in coronary artery disease was highlighted in Green's follow up report[82] on the original MRC trial in which propranolol, a diuretic and placebo were compared in middle-aged mildly hypertensive patients. Although the original paper showed that propranolol did not reduce coronary events significantly, Green showed that when silent infarct and sudden death were included, propranolol did significantly reduce coronary events. The MAPHY-HAPPHY study[83,84] was a controversial study in which initially metoprolol and diuretic treatments of moderately severe male hypertensives were compared. Subsequently, a parallel group was added in which atenolol and diuretics were compared. When the effects of both beta-blockers (metoprolol plus atenolol results) were compared with diuretics no difference was detected,[83,85] but when the effect of metoprolol alone and diuretics were compared it was evident that metoprolol significantly reduced total mortality, coronary mortality and sudden death.[84,86,87] Atenolol had been no more effective and was perhaps less effective than a diuretic.[85] Many found this difference between two selective beta-blockers inexplicable and unacceptable. However, the efficacy of metoprolol in reducing coronary mortality has been confirmed in post-MI studies[88–90] and in MERIT HF.[28] Atenolol's relative lack of effect on coronary events has also been confirmed.[79,91]

Post-MI trials

Randomized trials
The literature on beta-blockers in post-MI patients is now very extensive. Pooled data on over 25,000 patients in 24 trials revealed that mortality, cardiac death and sudden death were reduced by 21%, 24% and 30% respectively.[1] Sudden death and the importance of trying to reduce this mode of death in the management of heart failure deserve emphasis. Good data on this subject can be obtained from the timolol trial,[2] the BHAT propranolol trial,[3] and pooled data from several metoprolol trials,[89] which includes the Gothenburg

study.[88] Figure 1 shows the percentage of patients who died in each trial and the percentage who died suddenly. Overall, at least half of all those who die in the early years after a myocardial infarct die suddenly. The effect of the three beta-blockers on risk of sudden death is shown in Figure 2. No other class of drug has such a marked effect on sudden death associated with coronary artery disease, although ACE inhibitors do reduce the risk of sudden death.[92,93] The importance of this in relation to the management of heart failure is illustrated in Figure 3, which shows the figures for total deaths and sudden deaths side by side for each of the first three major heart failure studies.

Observational studies in at-risk patients
For many years, although many of the attributes of beta-blockers have been widely recognized, few patients who might have been helped have actually received them. This is because of the widespread belief, based on 1960s pharmacology that beta-blockers should not be given to the elderly,

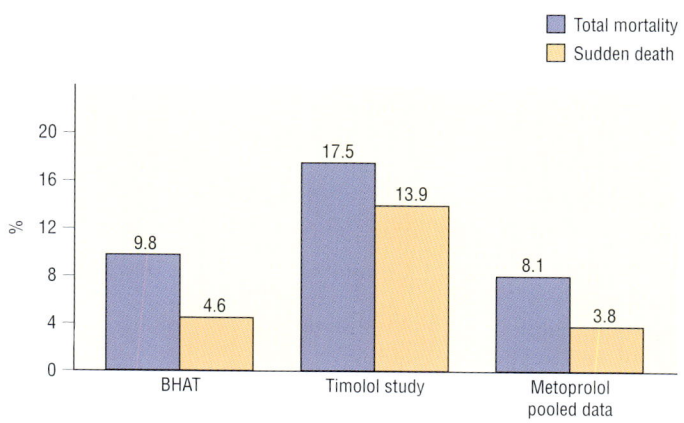

Figure 1
Total mortality and sudden death rates in three studies of beta-blockers in post-MI patients.[2,3,89]

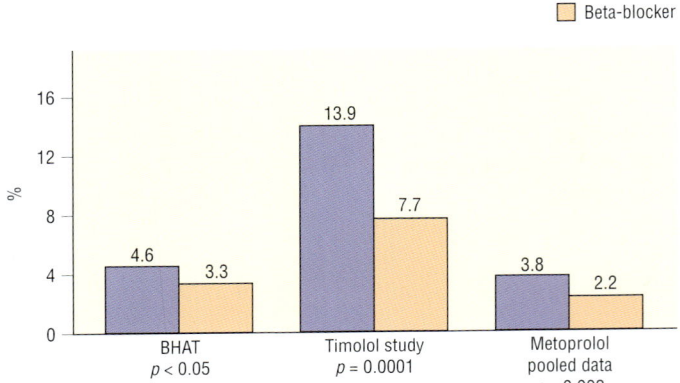

Figure 2
Impact of beta-blockers on sudden death in three post-MI studies[1,2,89]

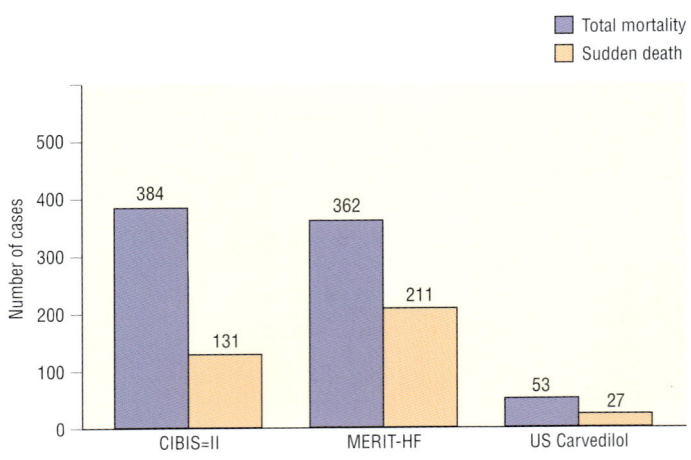

Figure 3
Total mortality and sudden death rates in three studies of beta-blockers in heart failure.[26,28,66]

or to people with asthma, diabetes or heart failure. Good clinical evidence suggests that, of these, only asthma remains as an absolute contraindication to the use of beta-blockers.

Some examples of the use of beta-blockers in the other at-risk groups show that they are relatively safe in the sort of people who might be given beta-blockers for heart failure. Furthermore, their cardioprotective effects are, if anything, more marked.

Elderly Soumerai and colleagues[94] reported in 1997 a retrospective study on drug use by elderly post-MI patients and its effect on survival. They identified 5332 patients aged 65 years or older who survived for 30 days after an acute MI. Of these, 3737 were judged eligible to receive beta-blockers. The main outcome was the use of beta-blockers and calcium channel blockers in the first 90 days after discharge, and mortality rates and readmissions to hospital with cardiac problems in the first 2 years after discharge. Only 21% of those eligible received a beta-blocker. Patients were three times more likely to receive a new prescription for a calcium channel blocker than for a beta-blocker. Controlling for other predictors of survival, those on a beta-blocker had a 43% lower mortality rate (relative risk, RR=0.57, 95% confidence interval 0.47–0.69). Beta-blockers were effective in all age groups, even in those over 85 years old (see Table 3). Use of a calcium channel

Table 3
Predictors of survival in those on a beta-blocker[94]

Age range (years)	Number of patients	Relative risk of death in those on a beta-blocker	95% confidence interval
65–74	1392	0.50	0.36–0.72
75–84	1744	0.56	0.43–0.73
85 and over	601	0.72	0.47–1.11

blocker instead of a beta-blocker was associated with twice the risk of death (RR = 1.98, 95% CI 1.44–2.72) "not because calcium channel blockers had demonstrable adverse effects but because they were substituted for beta-blockers".

The above study confirms the results in those aged 60–69 years in the beta-blocker heart attack trial (BHAT)[3] and in those aged 65–75 years in the Norwegian timolol study.[2] Further evidence that beta-blockers are well tolerated by elderly hypertensives was well provided by STOP-Hypertension[78] and STOP-2.[81]

Diabetes Diabetic patients are at risk of developing coronary artery disease[95] and may go on to develop heart failure. As a consequence, a fairly large number of patients with heart failure have diabetes.[96] Some data on the incidence of diabetes in well-known trials are presented in Table 4. Accordingly, it is important that a potential major treatment for heart failure should not be contraindicated in diabetes.

Experience in the major beta-blocker post-MI studies is now extensive and has been reviewed by Kjekshus and

Table 4
Incidence of diabetes mellitus in ACE inhibitor trials

Source	% Diabetic	Reference
Swedish Survey	10	Andersson et al, 1993[106]
CONSENSUS	23	Consensus, 1987[23]
SOLVD	25	SOLVD, 1991[107]
V-HEFT II	20	Cohn et al, 1991[108]
ATLAS	20	Massie et al, 1998[109]
RESOLVD	27	Suskin et al, 1998[110]

colleagues.[97] Evidence for the marked efficacy of beta-blockers is shown in Figure 4. An observational study of non-insulin dependent diabetes known to have coronary artery disease corroborated the observations of Kjekshus and colleagues.[97] It showed that 911 (33%) patients who were on a beta-blocker had a mortality rate of 7.8%, and 1812 patients who were not on a beta-blocker had a mortality rate of 14%.[98]

Malmberg and colleagues[99] have investigated the risk markers for mortality in diabetics with acute MI. They had already shown clearly the value of careful diabetic control at the time of an acute infarct. Table 5 shows some interesting associations and risk ratios based on 240 deaths, 138 (44%) in a control group (routine antidiabetic therapy) and 102 (33%) in an intensively treated group. Beta-blockers were associated with an overall 44% reduction in mortality, and the effect was greater in those whose diabetes was less well controlled.

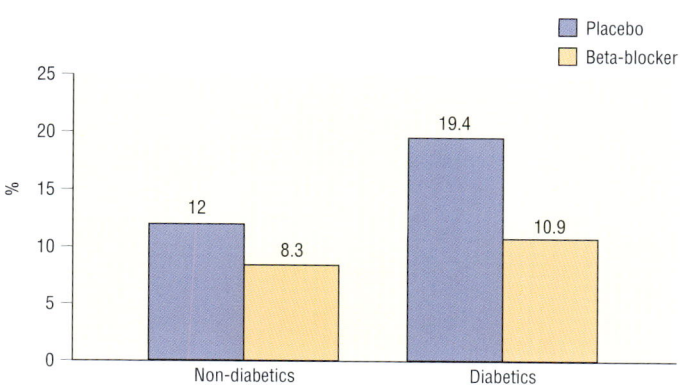

Figure 4
Impact of beta-blockers on diabetic and non-diabetic post-MI patients.[99]

Table 5

Univariate associations with long-term mortality in patients with diabetes mellitus and acute myocardial infarction – presented as relative risks

Parameter	All (n=620; deaths=240)		Patient groups Control[†] (n=314; deaths=138)		Intensively treated[††] (n=306; deaths=102)	
	RR*	p	RR*	p	RR*	p
Glycosylated haemoglobin	1.07	<0.05	1.13	<0.01	1.01	0.813
CCF in hospital	2.45	<0.001	2.59	<0.001	2.40	<0.001
Hospital thrombolysis	0.57	<0.001	0.69	<0.05	0.44	<0.001
β-blocker at discharge	0.56	<0.001	0.45	<0.001	0.69	0.097
ACE inhibitor at discharge	1.39	<0.05	1.46	0.053	1.35	0.179

*95% CI given in Table 3, reference 99.
[†]Routine antidiabetic therapy
[††]Insulin–glucose infusion

It is therefore apparent that diabetics benefit more from beta-blockers than non-diabetics. Data showing that patients with diabetes had an adverse effect from beta-blockers on diabetic control are more difficult to find.

High-risk patients Gottlieb and colleagues[100] analysed 201,752 post-MI patients aged over 65 years old. Their important study provides data on the efficacy and tolerability of beta-blockers in very large numbers of patients. Table 6 gives the numbers of patients in three of the many subgroups studied, namely the elderly, diabetics, and those with chronic obstructive pulmonary disease. The risk of death at 2 years is given in Table 7 and shown in Figures 5, 6, and 7. It is obvious that in these high-risk groups, beta-blockers have a very positive effect and are not harmful as pharmacologists used to predict.

Heart failure Until recently, heart failure was regarded as an absolute contraindication to beta-blockade. It was true, and still is true, that standard doses of beta-blockers given to a patient with heart failure may precipitate a rapid

Table 6
Number of patients assessed to determine the effect of beta-blockers (BB) on 2 year mortality in post-MI patients

Characteristic	Total number	Number on BB	Number not on BB
Age (years)			
<75	106,496	39,312	67,184
75–84	71,426	23,467	47,959
>85	23,830	6,374	17,456
Diabetes mellitus			
On Insulin	21,578	6,115	15,463
Not on Insulin	37,867	12,521	25,346
Prior COPD	41,814	9,228	32,586

Adapted from table 1, reference 100.

Table 7
Adjusted and relative risk of death at 2 years in post-MI patients on or not on beta-blockers (BB) at hospital discharge

Characteristic	Risk of death %		Relative risk (95% CI)
	on BB	Not on BB	
Age (years)			
<70	11.3	18.7	0.60 (0.57–0.63)
70–79	15.3	24.0	0.64 (0.58–0.70)
>80	22.6	33.1	0.68 (0.63–0.75)
Diabetes mellitus	17.0	26.6	0.64 (0.60–0.69)
Prior COPD	16.8	27.8	0.60 (0.57–0.63)

Adapted from table 2, reference 100.

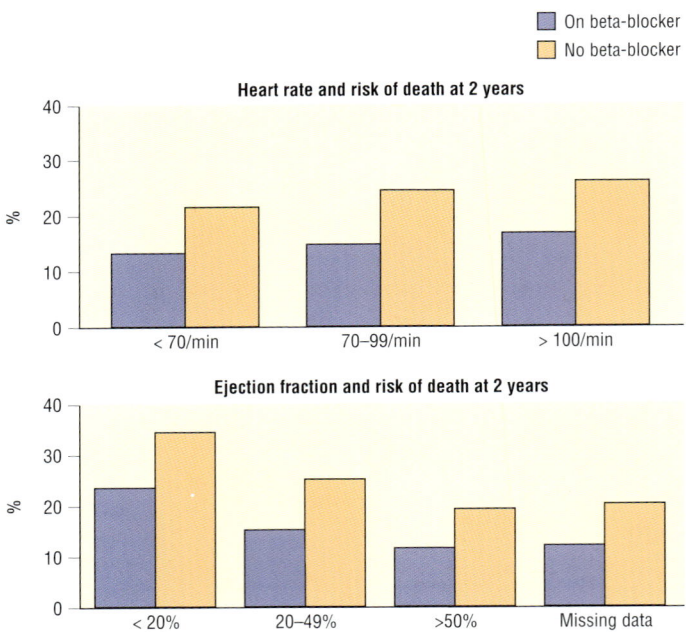

Figure 5
Impact of beta-blockers in post-MI patients with differing heart rates and ejection fractions.[100]

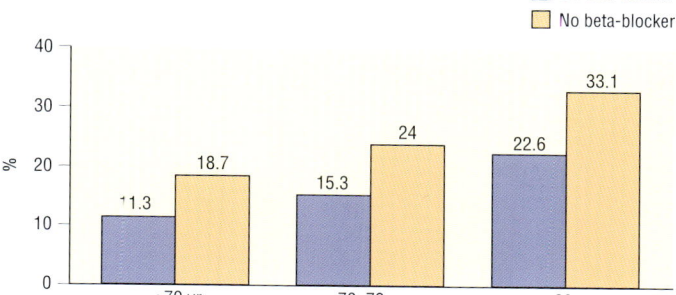

Figure 6

Impact of beta-blockers in post-MI in patients age <70, 70–79 and over 80 years old.[100]

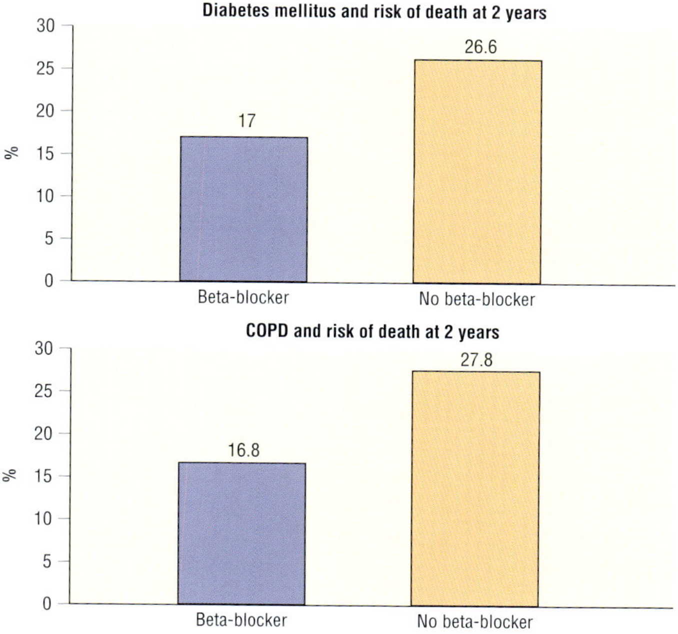

Diabetes mellitus and risk of death at 2 years

COPD and risk of death at 2 years

Figure 7

Impact of beta-blockers on post-MI patients with diabetes and patients with chronic obstructive pulmonary disease (COPD).

deterioration. The benefit from beta-blockade are obtained by stabilizing the patient first and using beta-blockers very cautiously, starting with a small dose and building up slowly.

Despite major concerns about the potential adverse effects of beta-blockers in patients with heart failure, there were quite large numbers of patients with heart failure in the post-MI studies. Results on those patients, for example the BHAT trial[3] and the Gothenburg trial,[90] indicated that beta-blockers were reasonably well tolerated and were effective. Houghton and colleagues[113] undertook a meta-analysis to determine the effect of beta-blockers in post-MI patients with heart failure or major cardiac dysfunction. They reviewed 17 trials, which included 20,333 patients of whom 1882 (9.3%) died. The analysis concluded that the effect of beta-blockers was similar in those with and without heart failure or ventricular dysfunction, but because those with heart failure are at great risk the absolute benefits of beta-blockers in this group are greater.

In the AIRE study, ramipril was assessed in post-MI patients with heart failure and those patients in this trial who were on a beta-blocker had a lower mortality (hazard ratio 0.66, 95% CI 0.40–0.83) and lower rate of progression to severe heart failure.[101] Finally, in the RALES trial those treated with beta-blockers appear to have benefited more.[102]

Trials of antiarrhythmic drugs Most trials of antiarrhythmic drugs in patients with coronary artery disease have failed to show a convincing beneficial effect on mortality. In fact, these drugs have tended to be associated with an increased mortality. However, in several trials, those patients who were also on a beta-blocker had a better prognosis. Table 8 presents data from CAST,[103] EMIAT,[104] and CAMIAT,[105] showing key results that suggest that being on a beta-blocker was beneficial. Furthermore, beta-blockers, specifically metoprolol CR/XL, have been shown

Table 8
Effect of beta-blockers in three antiarrhythmic drug trials in post-MI patients

	No beta-blockers	Beta-blockers
CAST study[103] Arrhythmic death or cardiac arrest at 2 years	14.7%	9.5%
EMIAT study[104] Relative Risk for Total Cardiac mortality (see fig 5, reference 104)	1.15	0.52
CAMIAT study[105] Resuscitated VF or arrhythmic death events (% rate/year)		
Amiodarone	13 (4.07)	2 (0.38)
Placebo	15 (4.03)	16 (2.93)

to help prevent relapse into atrial fibrillation or atrial flutter after cardioversion.[114]

Conclusions

In this chapter we have shown that:

- Beta-blockers work in several different ways that might benefit the patient with heart failure. The importance of slowing heart rate has been emphasized
- Animal data confirms the potential to reduce the risk of ventricular fibrillation
- Clinical data in hypertensive patients and post-MI patients have shown that beta-blockers reduce the risk of coronary events and sudden death. Data on timolol, propranolol and metoprolol are particularly persuasive
- Most patients, except asthmatics, tolerate and benefit from beta-blockers. Good data on the elderly, diabetic patients and those with heart failure are available.

Further, for carvedilol, bisoprolol, and metoprolol, the data for tolerability presented in this book are also very reassuring.

References

1. Freemantle N, Cleland J, Young P, Mason J, Harrison J. Beta-blockade after myocardial infarction: systematic review and meta regression analysis. *Br Med J* 1999; **318:** 1730–7.
2. The Norwegian Multicenter Study Group. Timolol-induced reduction in mortality and reinfarction in patients surviving acute myocardial infarction. *N Engl J Med* 1981; **304:** 801–7.
3. Beta-Blocker Heart Attack Research Group. A randomized trial of propranolol in patients with acute myocardial infarction. 1. Mortality results. *JAMA* 1982; **247:** 1707–14.
4. Packer M, Lee WH, Kessler PD, Gottlieb SS, Bernstein JL, Kukin MI. Role of neurohormonal mechanisms in determining survival in patients with severe chronic heart failure. *Circulation* 1987; **75** (suppl IV):80–92.
5. Chidsey CA, Harrison DC, Braunwald E. Augmentation of the plasma nor-epinephrine response to exercise in patients with congestive heart failure. *N Engl J Med* 1962; **267:** 650–4.
6. Thomas JA, Marks BH. Plasma norepinephrine in congestive heart failure. *Am J Cardiol* 1978; **41:** 233.
7. Cohn JN, Levine TB, Olivari MT, et al. Plasma norepinephrine as a guide to prognosis in patients with chronic congestive heart failure. *N Engl J Med* 1984; **311:** 819–23.
8. Dyer AR, Persky V, Stamler J, et al. Heart rate as a prognostic factor for coronary artery disease and mortality: findings in three Chicago epidemiologic studies. *Am J Epidemiol* 1980; **112:** 736–49.
9. Kannel WB, Kannel C, Paffenbarger-RS J, Cupples LA. Heart rate and cardiovascular mortality: the Framingham Study. *Am Heart J* 1987; **113:** 1489–94.
10. Gillum RF.The epidemiology of resting heart rate in a national sample of men and women: association with hypertension, coronary artery disease, blood pressure, and other cardiovascular risk factors. *Am Heart J* 1988; **116:** 163–74.
11. Gillum RF. Pulse rate, coronary artery disease, and death: the NHANES I Epidemiologic Follow-up Study. *Am Heart J* 1991; **121:** 172–7.
12. Shaper AG, Wannamethee G, Macfarlane PW, Walker M. Heart rate, ischaemic heart disease, and sudden cardiac death in middle-aged British men. *Br Heart J* 1993; **70:** 49–55.
13. Hjalmarson A, Gilpin E, Kjekshus J, et al. Influence of heart rate on mortality after acute myocardial infarction. *Am J Cardiol* 1990; **1:** 547–53.

14. Moser DK. Stevenson WG, Woo MA, Stevenson LW. Timing of sudden death in patients with heart failure. *J Am Coll Cardiol* 1994; **24:** 963–7.

15. ISIS-2 collaborative group (Second International Study of Infarct Survival). Morning peak in the incidence of myocardial infarction: experience in the ISIS-2 trial. *Eur Heart J* 1992; **13:** 594–8.

16. Beere PA, Glasgow S, Zarins CK. Retarding effect of lowered heart rate on coronary atherosclerosis. *Science* 1984; **226:** 180–2.

17. Waagstein F, Caidahl K, Wallentin I, Bergh CH, Hjalmarson A. Long term beta-blockade in dilated cardiomyopathy: effects of short and long-term metoprolol treatment followed by withdrawal and readministration of metoprolol. *Circulation* 1989; **90:** 551–63.

18. Kjekshus JK, Blix AS, Grottum P, Aasen AO. Beneficial effects of vagal stimulation on the ischaemic myocardium during beta-receptor blockade. *Scand J Clin Lab Invest* 1981; **41:** 383–9.

19. Kjekshus J, Gullestad L. Heart rate as a therapeutic target in heart failure. *Eur Heart J* 1999; **1**(suppl H): H64–H69.

20. International Collaborative Study Group. Reduction in infarct size with the early use of timolol in acute myocardial infarction. *N Engl J Med* 1984; **310:** 9–15.

21. Kjekshus J. Importance of heart rate in determining beta-blocker efficacy in acute and long-term acute myocardial infarction intervention trials. *Am J Cardiol* 1986; **57:** 43f–49f.

22. St John Sutton M, Pfeffer MA, Moye L. Cardiovascular death and left ventricular remodelling two years after myocardial infarction. Baseline predictor and impact of long-term use of Captopril: information from the survival and ventricular enlargement (SAVE) trial. *Circulation* 1997; **96:** 3294–9.

23. Swedberg K, Eneroth P, Kjekshus J, Wilhelmsen L. The Consensus Trial Study Group. Hormone regulation of cardiovascular function in patients with severe congestive heart failure and the relation to mortality. *Circulation* 1990; **82:** 1730–7.

24. Nul DR, Doval HC, Grancelli HO. Heart rate is a marker of amiodarone mortality reduction in severe heart failure. *J Am Coll Cardiol* 1997; **29:** 1199–205.

25. CIBIS Investigators and Committees. A randomized trial of beta-blockade in heart failure. *Circulation* 1994; **90:** 1765–73.

26. CIBIS-II Investigators and Committees. The cardiac insufficiency bisoprolol study II (CIBIS-II): a randomised trial. *Lancet* 1999; **353:** 9–13.

27. BEST Steering Committee. Design of the Beta-blocker Evaluation of Survival Trial (BEST). *Am J Cardiol* 1995; **75:** 1220–3.

28. MERIT-HF Study Group. Effect of metoprolol CR/XL in chronic heart failure: metoprolol CR/XL randomised intervention trial in congestive heart failure (MERIT-HF). *Lancet* 1999; **353:** 2001–7.

29. Lechat P, Escolano S, Golmard JL, et al. Prognostic value of bisoprolol induced hemodynamic effects in heart failure during the Cardiac Insufficiency Bisoprolol Study (CIBIS). *Circulation* 1997; **96:** 2197–205.

30. Saul JP, Arai Y, Berger RD, Lilly LS, Colucci WS, Cohen RJ. Assessment of autonomic regulation in chronic congestive heart failure by heart rate spectral analysis. *Am J Cardiol* 1988; **61:** 1292–99.

31. Casolo G, Balli E, Taddei T, Amumasi J, Gori C. Decreased spontaneous heart rate variability in congestive heart failure. *Am J Cardiol* 1989; **64:** 1162–7.

32. Kleiger RE, Miller JP, Bigger JT, Moss AJ. Decreased heart rate variability and its association with increased mortality after myocardial infarction. *Am J Cardiol* 1987; **59:** 256–62.

33. Cook JR, Bigger JT, Kleiger RE, Fleiss JL, Steinman AB, Rolnitzky LM. Effect of atenolol and diltiazem on heart period variability in normal persons. *J Am Coll Cardiol* 1991; **17:** 480–4.

34. Molgaard H, Mickley H, Pless P, Bjerregaard P, Moller M. Effects of metoprolol on heart rate variability in survivors of acute myocardial infarction. *Am J Cardiol* 1993; **71:** 1357–9.

35. Coumel P, Hermida JS, Wennerblom B, Leenhardt A, Maison-Blanche P, Cauchemez B. Heart rate variability in left ventricular hypertrophy and heart failure, and the effects of beta-blockade. *Eur Heart J* 1991; **12:** 412–22.

36. Niemelä MJ, Airakasinen KEJ, Huikuri H. Effect of beta-blockade on heart rate variability in patients with coronary artery disease. *J Am Coll Cardiol* 1994; **23:** 1370–7.

37. Andersson B, Strömblad SO, Lomsky M, Waagstein F. Heart rate dependency of cardiac performance in heart failure patients treated with metoprolol. *Eur Heart J* 1999; **20:** 575–83.

38. Lechat PP, Packer M, Chalon S, et al. Clinical effects of beta adrenergic blockade in chronic heart failure: a meta analysis of double blind, placebo controlled randomised trials. *Circulation* 1998; **98:** 1184–91.

39. Doughty RN, Whalley GA, Gamble G, and the Australian/New Zealand Heart Failure Research Collaborative Group. Left ventricular remodelling with carvedilol in patients with congestive heart failure due to ischaemic heart disease. *J Am Coll Cardiol* 1997; **29:** 1060–6.

40. Andersson B, Caidahl K, Waagstein F. Recovery from left ventricular asynergy in ischemic cardiomyopathy following long-term beta blockade treatment. *Cardiology* 1994; **85:** 14–22.

41. Ng KS, Gibson DG. Impairment of diastolic function by shortened filling period in severe left ventricular disease. *Br Heart J* 1989; **62:** 246–52.

42. Eichorn EJ, Bristow MR. Medical therapy can improve the biological properties of the chronically failing heart: a new era in the treatment of heart failure. *Circulation* 1996; **94:** 2285–96.

43. Colucci WS. Molecular and cellular mechanisms of myocardial failure. *Am J Cardiol* 1997; **80:** 15L–25L.

44. Metra M, Nodari S, D'Aloia A. A rationale for the use of beta-blockers as standard treatment for heart failure. *Am Heart J* 2000; **139:** 511–21.
45. Podrid PJ, Fuchs T, Candinas R. Role of the sympathetic nervous system in the genesis of ventricular arrhythmia. *Circulation* 1990; **82:** 1103–13.
46. Parker GW, Michael LH, Hartley CJ, Skinner JE, Entman MC. Central beta-adrenergic mechanisms may modulate ischemic ventricular fibrillation in pigs. *Circ Res* 1990; **66:** 259–70.
47. Delsperger KC, Martins JB, Clothier JL, Marcus ML. Incidence of sudden cardiac death associated with coronary artery occlusion in dogs with hypertension and left ventricular hypertrophy is reduced by chronic beta-adrenergic blockade. *Circulation* 1990; **82:** 941–50.
48. Ablad B. Bjuro T, Bjorkman JA, Edstrom T, Olsson G. Role of central nervous beta-adrenoceptors in the prevention of ventricular fibrillation through the augmentation of cardiac vagal tone. *J Am Coll Cardiol* 1991; **17:** 165A.
49. Yates VC, Beamish RE, Dhalla NS. Ventricular dysfunction and necrosis produced by adrenochrome metabolite of epinephrine: relation to pathogenesis of catecholamine cardiomyopathy. *Am Heart J* 1981; **102:** 210–21.
50. Lowe MC, Reinchenbach DD. Pharmacological and morphological aspects of the isoproterenol induced lesion in the rat Langendorff heart. *Proc West Pharmacol Soc* 1977; **20:** 419–20.
51. Haft JI. Cardiovascular injury induced by sympathetic catecholamines. *Prog Cardiovasc Dis* 1974; **17:** 73–86.
52. Katz A. Cellular mechanisms in congestive heart failure. *Am J Cardiol* 1988; **62:** 3A–8A.
53. Sharov VG, Sabbah HN, Shimoyama H, Goussev AV, Lesch M, Goldstein S. Evidence of cardiocyte apoptosis in myocardium of dogs with chronic heart failure. *Am J Pathol* 1996; **148:** 141–9.
54. Sabbah HN, Sharov VG. Apoptosis in heart failure. *Prog Cardiovasc Dis* 1988; **40:** 549–62.
55. Sabbah HN. The cellular and physiologic effects of beta blockers in heart failure. *Clin Cardiol* 1999; **22** (Suppl V): V16–V20.
56. Sabbah HN, Sharon VG, Goussev A. Long term therapy with metoprolol attenuates cardiomyocyte apoptosis in dogs with heart failure. *Circulation* 1988; **98** (suppl 1): 364.
57. Eichhorn EJ, Heesch CM, Barnett JH, et al. Effect of metoprolol on myocardial function and energetics in patients with non ischemic dilated cardiomyopathy: a randomized, double-blind, placebo controlled study. *J Am Coll Cardiol* 1994; **24:** 1310–20.
58. Jewett SL, Eddy LJ, Hochstein P. Is the autoxidation of catecholamines involved in ischemia-reperfusion injury? *Free Radical Biol Med* 1999; **6:** 185–8.
59. Kukin ML, Kalman J, Charney RH, et al. Prospective, randomised comparison of effect of long-term treatment with metoprolol or

carvedilol on symptoms, exercise, ejection fraction, and oxidative stress in heart failure. *Circulation* 1999; **99:** 2645–51.

60. Belch JF, Bridges AB, Scott N, Chopra M. Oxygen free radicals and congestive heart failure. *Br Heart J* 1991; **65:** 245–8.

61. McMurray J, McLay J, Chopra MB, Bridges A, Belch JF. Evidence for enhanced free radical activity in chronic congestive heart failure secondary to coronary artery disease. *Am J Cardiol* 1990; **65:** 1261–2.

62. McMurray J, Chopra MB, Abdullah I, Smith WE, Dargie HJ. Evidence of oxidative stress in chronic heart failure in humans. *Eur Heart J* 1993; **14:** 1493–8.

63. Ferrari R, Agnoletti L, Comini L, et al. Oxidative stress during myocardial ischaemia and heart failure. *Eur Heart J* 1998; **19** (suppl B): B2–B11.

64. Yue T-L, Cheng H-Y, Lysko PG, et al. Carvedilol, a new vasodilator and beta adrenoceptor antagonist, is an antioxidant and free radical scavenger. *J Pharmacol Exper Therapeutics* 1992; **263:** 92–8.

65. Lopez BL, Christopher TA, Yue T-L, Ruffolo R, Feuerstein GZ, Ma X-L. Carvedilol, a new beta-adrenoreceptor blocker antihypertensive drug, protects against free-radical-induced endothelial dysfunction. *Pharmacology* 1995; **51:**165–73.

66. Packer M, Bristow MR, Cohn JN, et al, and the US Carvedilol Heart Failure Study Group (1996) The effect of carvedilol on morbidity and mortality in patients with chronic heart failure. *N Engl J Med* 1996; **334:** 1349–55.

67. Thubrikar MJ, Christie AM, Cao-Danh HC, Holloway PE, Nolan SP. Metoprolol reduces low density lipoprotein uptake in aortic regions prone to atherosclerosis. *FASEB J* 1990; **4:** A1151.

68. Kaplan JR, Manuck SB, Adams MR, Weingand KW, Clarkson TB. Inhibition of coronary atherosclerosis by propranolol in behaviourally predisposed monkeys fed an atherogenic diet. *Circulation* 1987; **76:** 1364–72.

69. Kaplan Jr, Manuck S, Adams M, Clarkson T. The effects of beta-adrenergic blocking agents on atherosclerosis and its complications. *Eur Heart J* 1987; **8:** 929–44.

70. Strawn W, Bondjers G, Kaplan JR, et al. Endothelial dysfunction in response to psychosocial stress in monkeys. *Circ Res* 1991; **68:** 1270–9.

71. Spence JD, Perkins DG, Klein RL, Adams MR, Haust MD. Haemodynamic modifications of aortic atherosclerosis: effects of propranolol versus hydralazine in hypertensive hyperlipidaemic rabbits. *Atherosclerosis* 1984; **50:** 325–33.

72. Linden T, Camejo G, Wiklund O, Warnold I, Olofsson SO, Bondjers G. Effect of short-term beta blockade on serum lipid levels and on the interaction of LDL with human arterial proteoglycans. *J Clin Pharmacol* 1990; **30:** S123–S131.

73. Frishman WH, Christodoulou J, Weksler B, et al. Abrupt propranolol withdrawal in angina pectoris: effects on platelet aggregation and exercise tolerance. *Am Heart J* 1978; **95:** 169–79.

74. Willich SN, Pohjola-Sintonen S, Bhatia SH, et al. Suppression of silent ischaemia by metoprolol without alteration of morning increase of platelet aggregability in patients with stable coronary artery disease. *Circulation* 1989; **79:** 557–65.

75. Ablad B, Bjorkman JA, Gustafsson D, et al. The role of sympathetic activity in atherogenesis: effects of beta-blockade. *Am Heart J* 1988; **116:** 322–7.

76. Hedblad B, Wikstrand J, Janzon L, Wedel H, Berglund G. Low-dose metoprolol CR/XL and fluvastatin slow progression of carotid intima-media thickness. Main results from the beta-blocker Cholesterol-Lowering Asymptomatic Plaque Study (BCAPS). *Circulation* 2001; **103:** 1721–6.

77. SHEP Cooperative Research Group. Prevention of stroke by antihypertensive drug treatment in older persons with isolated systolic hypertension. *JAMA* 1991; **265:** 3255–64.

78. Dahlöf B, Lindholm LH, Hansson L, Scherstén B, Ekbom T, Wester PO. Morbidity and mortality in the Swedish Trial in old patients with hypertension (STOP-Hypertension). *Lancet* 1991; **338:** 1281–5.

79. MRC Working Party. Medical Research Council trial of treatment of hypertension in older adults: Principal results. *Br Med J* 1992; **304:** 405–12.

80. Staessen JA, Fagard R, Thijs L, et al. Randomised double-blind comparison of placebo and active treatment for older patients with isolated systolic hypertension. *Lancet* 1997; **350:** 757–64.

81. Hansson L, Lindholm LH, Ekbom T, et al, and the STOP-Hypertension 2 Study Group. Comparison of "old" versus "newer" antihypertensive therapies in preventing cardiovascular mortality and morbidity in elderly hypertensives: principal results of the Swedish trial in old patients with hypertension-2 (STOP-Hypertension-2). *Lancet* 1999; **354:** 1751–6.

82. Green KG. British MRC trial of treatment for mild hypertension – a more favourable interpretation. *Am J Hypertens* 1991; **4:** 723–4.

83. Wilhelmsen L, Berglund G, Elmfeldt D, et al. Beta-blockers versus diuretics in hypertensive men: main results from the HAPPHY trial. *J Hypertens* 1987; **5:** 561–72.

84. Wikstrand J, Warnold I, Olsson G, Toumilehto J, Elmfeldt D, Berglund G. Primary prevention with metoprolol in patients with hypertension. Mortality results from the MAPHY study. *JAMA* 1988; **259:** 1976–82.

85. Holme I. MAPHY and the two arms of HAPPHY. *JAMA* 1989; **262:** 3272–4.

86. Olsson G, Tuomilehto J, Berglund G, et al. Primary prevention of sudden cardiovascular death in hypertensive patients: mortality results from the MAPHY study. *Am J Hypertens* 1991; **4:** 151–8.

87. Kendall MJ, Lynch KP, Hjalmarson A, Kjekshus J. Beta-blockers and sudden cardiac death. *Ann Intern Med* 1995; **123:** 358–67.
88. Hjalmarson A, Elmfeldt D, Herlitz J, et al. Effect on mortality of metoprolol in acute myocardial infarction. *Lancet* 1981; **ii:** 823–7.
89. Olsson G, Wikstrand J, Warnold I, et al. Metoprolol-induced reduction in postinfarction mortality: pooled results from five double-blind randomized trials. *Eur Heart J* 1992; **13:** 28–32.
90. Herlitz J, Waagstein F, Lindqvist J, Swedberg K. Effect of metoprolol on the prognosis for patients with suspected acute myocardial infarction and indirect signs of congestive heart failure (A subgroup analysis of the Göteborg metoprolol trial). *Am J Cardiol* 1997; **80**(9B): 40J–44J.
91. Coope J, Warrender TS. Randomised trial of treatment of hypertension in elderly patients in primary care. *BMJ* 1986; **293:** 1145–51.
92. Kober L, Torp-Pedersen C, Carlsen JE, et al, and the Trandolapril Cardiac Evaluation (TRACE) Study group. A clinical trial of the Angiotensin-converting enzyme inhibitor trandolapril in patients with left ventricular dysfunction after myocardial infarction. *N Engl J Med* 1995; **333:** 1670–6.
93. Cleland JGF, Erhardt L, Murray G, Hall AS, Ball SG, and the AIRE Study Investigators. Effect of ramipril on morbidity and mode of death among survivors of acute myocardial infarction with clinical evidence of heart failure. *Eur Heart J* 1997; **18:** 41–51.
94. Soumerai S, McLaughlin T, Spiegelman D, Hertzmarck E, Thibault G, Goldman L. Adverse outcomes of underuse of beta-blockers in elderly survivors of acute myocardial infarction. *JAMA* 1997; **277:** 115–21.
95. Haffner S, Lehto S, Ronnemaa T, Pyorala K, Laakso M. Mortality from coronary heart disease in subjects with Type 2 diabetes and in nondiabetic subjects with and without prior myocardial infarction. *N Engl J Med* 1998; **339:** 229–34.
96. Soläng L, Malmberg K, Rydén L. Diabetes mellitus and congestive heart failure. *Eur Heart J* 1999; **20:** 789–95.
97. Kjekshus J, Gilpin J, Cali G, et al. Diabetic patients and beta-blockers after acute myocardial infarction. *Eur Heart J* 1990; **11:** 43–50.
98. Jonas M, Reicher-Reiss H, Boyko V, et al. Usefulness of beta-blocker therapy in patients with non-insulin dependent diabetes mellitus and coronary artery disease. *Am J Cardiol* 1996; **77:** 1273–7.
99. Malmberg K, Norhammar A, Wedel H, Rydén L. Glycometabolic state at admission: important risk marker of mortality in conventionally treated patients with diabetes mellitus and acute myocardial infarction. *Circulation* 1999; **99:** 2626–32.
100. Gottlieb S, McCarter R, Vogel RA. Effect of Beta-blockade on mortality among high-risk and low-risk patients after myocardial infarction. *N Engl J Med* 1988; **339:** 489–97.
101. Spargias KS, Hall AS, Greenwood DC, Ball SG. Beta-blocker treatment and other prognostic variables in patients with clinical

evidence of heart failure after acute myocardial infarction: evidence from the AIRE study. *Heart* 1999; **81:** 25–32.

102. Pitt B, Zannad F, Remme WJ, et al, and the Randomized Aldactone evaluation study investigators. The effect of spironolactone on morbidity and mortality in patients with severe heart failure. *N Engl J Med* 1999; **341:** 709–17.

103. Kennedy H, Brooks MM, Barker A, et al, and the CAST Investigators. Beta-blocker therapy in the cardiac arrhythmia suppression trial. *Am J Cardiol* 1994; **74:** 674–80.

104. Julian DG, Camm AJ, Frangin G, et al. Randomised trial of effect of amiodarone on mortality in patients with left-ventricular dysfunction after recent myocardial infarction: EMIAT. *Lancet* 1997; **349:** 667–74.

105. Cairns JA, Connolly SJ, Roberts R, Gent M. Randomised trial of outcome after myocardial infarction in patients with frequent or repetitive ventricular premature depolarisations: CAMIAT. *Lancet* 1997; **349:** 675–82.

106. Andersson B, Waagstein F. Spectrum and outcome of congestive heart failure in a hospitalised population. *Am Heart J* 1993; **126:** 632–40.

107. The SOLVD Investigators. Effect of enalapril on mortality and development of heart failure in asymptomatic patients with reduced left ventricular ejection fractions and congestive heart failure. *N Engl J Med* 1992; **327:** 685–91.

108. Cohn JN, Johnson G, Ziesche S, et al. A comparison of enalapril with hydralazine-isosorbide dinitrate in the treatment of chronic congestive heart failure. *N Engl J Med* 1991; **325:** 303–10.

109. Massie BM, Cleland JG, Armstrong PW, Packer M, Poole-Wilson PA, Lars R. Regional differences in the characteristics and treatment of patients participating in an international heart failure trial. The Assessment of Treatment with Lisinopril and Survival (ATLAS) Trial Investigators. *J Cardiac Failure* 1998; **4**(1): 3–8.

110. Suskin N, McKelvie RS, Roteau J, Sigouin C, Wiece KE, Yusuf S. Increased insulin and glucose levels in heart failure. *J Am Coll Cardiol* 1998; **3**(Suppl): 249A.

111. Gillman MW, Kannel WB, Belanger A, Dagostino RB. Influence of heart rate on mortality among persons with hypertension: The Framingham Study. *Am Heart J* 1993; **125:** 1148–54.

112. Gunderson T, Grottum P, Pedersen T, Kjekshus JK. Effect of timolol on mortality and reinfarction after acute myocardial infarction: prognostic importance of heart rate at rest. *Am J Cardiol* 1996; **58:** 20–4.

113. Houghton T, Freemantle N, Cleland JGF. Are beta-blockers effective in patients who develop heart failure soon after myocardial infarction? A meta-regression analysis of randomised trials. *Eur J Heart Failure* 2000; **2:** 333–40.

114. Kuhlkamp V, Schirdewan A, Stangl A, et al. Use of metoprolol CR/XL to maintain sinus rhythm after conversion from persistent atrial fibrillation: a randomised, double-blind, placebo-controlled study. *J Am Coll Cardiol* 2000; **36:** 139–46.

Carvedilol

Carvedilol is a non-selective beta-receptor antagonist. It also blocks alpha receptors[1] and has antioxidant properties, though the relevance of these ancillary properties is uncertain.[2] Alpha-blockers have not found a role in the management of heart failure, and in one study metoprolol was shown to have similar antioxidant properties.[3] Carvedilol was approved in the USA for treatment of hypertension in September 1995, and in May 1997 was the first beta-blocker to be given approval for the treatment of heart failure. It has been shown to relieve symptoms in angina and has recently been shown to reduce mortality and the rate of re-infarction in high-risk post-MI patients.

The clinical effects of carvedilol in heart failure have been shown in three clinical trials. The first of these, the US Carvedilol Programme (USCP) reported in the *New England Journal of Medicine*,[4] was relatively large, and suggested that carvedilol might reduce mortality from heart failure. The second, the Australian/New Zealand Heart Failure Study,[5] provided good supportive evidence for the efficacy of carvedilol in heart failure but was not large enough to give meaningful data on mortality. The third and definitive trial with carvedilol, the Carvedilol Prospective Randomised Cumulative Survival (COPERNICUS) trial, clearly showed that carvedilol improves survival in patients with severe heart failure. The USCP and COPERNICUS are described and discussed in this chapter.

The US carvedilol programme (USCP)

Four trials were undertaken to assess the effect of carvedilol in heart failure, and a prospectively defined over-all objective of the programme was to assess the effect of the drug on survival.[4]

Patients and methods

All patients had symptoms of heart failure for at least 3 months, an ejection fraction of 35% or less despite at least two months treatment with diuretics and, if tolerated, ACE inhibitors. Patients were excluded if they had had a major cardiovascular event recently, if they had had surgery within 3 months, or if they had myocarditis, uncorrected valvular disease or severe arrhythmias. As part of their ini-tial assessment patients had a 6-minute corridor walk test, and on the basis of the distance walked they were divided into four groups. The key features of the four component trials included in USCP are shown in Figure 8. The end-points of each of the four components are presented in Table 9.

All patients had a 2-week trial period of carvedilol 6.25 mg twice daily, a dose which could be halved temporarily if necessary. Those who tolerated the full dose were then randomly assigned carvedilol or placebo in the ratio 2:1 for mild and severe heart failure and 1:1 for moderate heart failure. After the two-week trial period the starting dose was 12.5 mg twice daily and this was increased to 25 mg and then 50 mg twice daily, if tolerated. Patients in the dose-ranging study were allocated to four parallel treat-ment groups, which were given placebo, or carvedilol 6.25 mg, 12.5 mg or 25 mg twice daily. All these studies were amalgamated and the results presented as if it was all one trial.

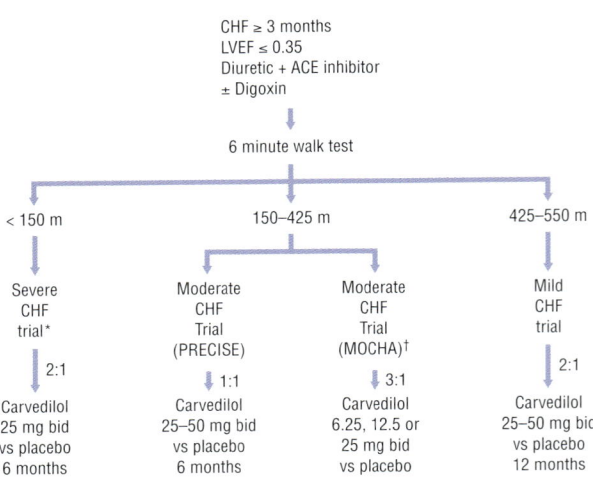

CHF ≥ 3 months
LVEF ≤ 0.35
Diuretic + ACE inhibitor
± Digoxin

6 minute walk test

< 150 m	150–425 m		425–550 m
Severe CHF trial*	Moderate CHF Trial (PRECISE)	Moderate CHF Trial (MOCHA)†	Mild CHF trial
2:1	1:1	3:1	2:1
Carvedilol 25 mg bid vs placebo 6 months	Carvedilol 25–50 mg bid vs placebo 6 months	Carvedilol 6.25, 12.5 or 25 mg bid vs placebo	Carvedilol 25–50 mg bid vs placebo 12 months

*Neither enrolment nor follow-up completed by time US carvedilol programme stopped.
†Dose response study.

Figure 8
Design of USCP trials in CHF.

Table 9
Endpoints of component trials on USCP

Trial	Primary endpoint	Other endpoints
Mild	Progression of CHF	LVEF*, NYHA class*, HF Score*, global assessment*, QoL, 9 min SPT, heart size on CXR, death*
Moderate (MOCHA)	6 min walk 9 min SPT	LVEF*, CHF hospital admission, (QoL, global assessment, death*)
Moderate (PRECISE)	6 min walk 9 min SPT	Global assessment*, NYHA Class*, LVEF*, QoL, CV hospital admission
Severe	QoL	Death, CV hospital admission, global assessment*, NYHA class, LVEF*, 6 min walk

*Significant, between group, difference. CV = cardiovascular; CXR = chest radiography; HF = heart failure score; QoL = quality of life; SPT = self-powered treadmill

Aim of study

The individual component trials had varying primary and secondary endpoints. However, a prospective pooling of deaths in all four trials was planned because of concerns that new drugs for CHF can increase mortality. The USCP, therefore, set out to recruit a sufficient number of patients to rule out (with 95% confidence) a 33% increase in the risk of death with carvedilol, compared with placebo (assuming an annual mortality rate of 12%). Because it was recognised that carvedilol might also reduce mortality, all statistical analyses were two sided. No formal stopping rules had been drawn up for the programme.

Results

Details of the USCP are presented in Figure 8. After randomization the patients received a total daily dose of 45 ± 27mg carvedilol. The median follow up was 6.5 months and no patients were lost to follow-up. The mortality rates were 31 (7.8%) on placebo and 22 (3.6%) on carvedilol – a highly significant difference ($p < 0.001$, Figure 9). The mode of death in each group is also shown.

The number of patients admitted to hospital at least once for cardiovascular reasons was 98 (14.1%) in the carvedilol group and 78 (19.6%) in the placebo group.

Detailed evaluation of the USCP

In this section, the design and results of the USCP studies are compared with CIBIS-II[6] and MERIT-HF,[7] details of which are given in subsequent chapters. Details of the design and conduct of the major beta-blocker heart failure trials are presented in Appendix Table A1, and the inclusion criteria in Appendix Table A2.

The USCP trials differed in three fundamental ways from CIBIS-II and MERIT-HF:

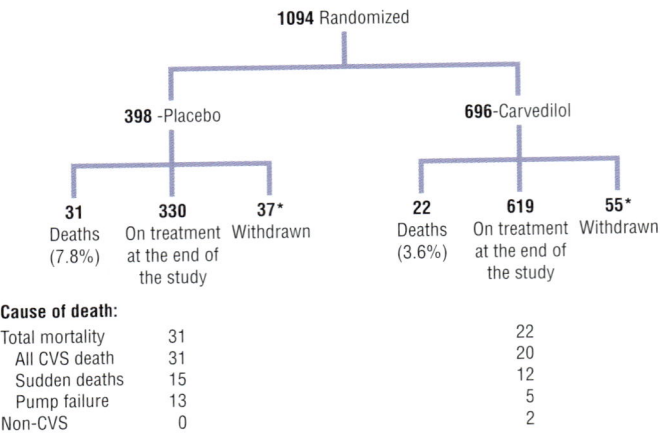

	1094 Randomized	
398 -Placebo		**696**-Carvedilol

| **31** Deaths (7.8%) | **330** On treatment at the end of the study | **37*** Withdrawn | | **22** Deaths (3.6%) | **619** On treatment at the end of the study | **55*** Withdrawn |

Cause of death:		
Total mortality	31	22
All CVS death	31	20
Sudden deaths	15	12
Pump failure	13	5
Non-CVS	0	2

*These figures were derived by subtracting the numbers dying plus those still on treatment from the total number entered.

Figure 9
USCP trial profile.

1. In the USCP trials patients had to undergo an "open-label" run-in phase in which they received unblinded carvedilol therapy for 2 weeks. Only patients tolerating 6.25 mg of carvedilol twice daily were eligible for randomization. This approach excluded patients unable to tolerate beta-blocker treatment and is controversial. It makes it difficult to analyse events occurring during the run-in phase, to assess adverse event rates, and to determine the proportion of patients achieving the target dose of test drug (see below). CIBIS-II and MERIT-HF did not have a run-in phase.
2. All patients in the USCP undertook a baseline exercise test to determine which component trial the patient entered.
3. Twice as many patients were randomized to carvedilol as to placebo.

Details of patients

The total number of patients recruited in the USCP was much smaller than in the other two trials, and they differed from those in the other trials in several ways (Appendix Table A3):

1. Their mean age was only 58 years.
2. The average left ventricular ejection fraction (LVEF) was much (5 percentage points) lower than in CIBIS-II and MERIT-HF.
3. Mean systolic blood pressure was 15 mm Hg lower than in the other two trials.

Overall, this suggests the USCP patients should have been sicker, higher risk patients, yet more were classed as NYHA Class II patients than in the other trials (see "event rates" below). A much higher proportion (30–40% more) of USCP patients received digoxin than in CIBIS-II or MERIT-HF. The significance of this difference is unclear but it could be important and has been generally overlooked. Concomitant medication is given in Appendix Table A4.

Event rates

It is very difficult to compare event rates in the USCP trials to those in CIBIS-II and MERIT-HF because of the very short (median 6.5 months) follow-up and the very small number of events in the USCP (Appendix Table A5, and Tables 10 and 11). The reported placebo group mortality at 6 months was 7.8% and the survival curves suggest an annual mortality rate of 10–11%, ie approaching that of MERIT-HF. The event rates in USCP do, however, seem similar to those in previous trials. The 6-month mortality rate in the enalapril group of SOLVD-T was 7.1%; the rate at 1 year was 12.3%.[8] The 6-month mortality rate in NET-WORK was, however, only 3.5%[9] and the 1-year rate in the captopril group of ELITE-I, which randomly assigned elderly patients, was 8.7%.[10]

Table 10
Effect of placebo and carvedilol treatment on mortality in patient sub-groups

| Variable * | Deaths (n)/patients(n) | | Hazard ratio (95% CI) |
	Placebo	Carvedilol	
Protocol			
Mild heart failure	5/134 (4%)	2/232 (1%)	0.22 (0.04–1.14)
Moderate heart failure	11/145 (8%)	6/133 (4%)	0.57 (0.21–1 54)
Moderate heart failure	13/84 (15%)	12/261 (5%)	0.27 (0.12–0.60)
Severe heart failure	2/35 (6%)	2/70 (3%)	0.53 (0.07–3.76)
LVEF			
< 0.23	20/209 (10%)	10/334 (4%)	0.25 (0.11–0.56)
> 0.23	11/189 (6%)	12/360 (3%)	0.49 (0.21–1.14)
Cause of heart failure			
Ischaemic	17/189 (9%)	13/332 (4%)	0.35 (0.16–0.73)
Non-ischaemic	14/208 (7%)	9/362 (3%)	0.35 (0.15–0.83)
NYHA Class			
Class II	12/108 (6%)	9/374 (2%)	0.40 (0.17–0.94)
Class III	19/177 (11%)	11/303 (4%)	0.33 (0.16–0.70)
Class IV	0/13 (0%)	2/19 (11%)	†

CI = Confidence interval; NYHA = New York Heart Association.
*For ejection fraction, medians were used to define the sub-groups.
The course of heart failure was not recorded for one patient in the
placebo group and two in the carvedilol group. The ejection fraction
was not recorded for two patients in the carvedilol group.
†Not calculable for NYHA Class IV.

Table 11
Hospital admissions in the USCP

Cause	Placebo	Carvedilol	*p* value
% Patients admitted			
Any cause	27	19	0.009
Cardiovascular	19.6	14.1	0.034
Heart failure	9	6	0.041
Number of admissions			
Any cause	160	208	0.003
Cardiovascular	119	143	0.021
Heart failure	61	52	0.028

In the placebo group of the USCP, 19.6% of patients had at least one hospital admission for a cardiovascular reason; the proportion admitted to hospital for any reason was 27% and for heart failure it was 9% (Table 11). The proportions in ELITE-I admitted for any reasons and for heart failure were 22.2% and 5.7% respectively.[10] The proportion of NETWORK patients requiring hospital admission related to heart failure was 5.1%.[9] Overall these comparisons suggest that the patients randomly assigned treatment in the USCP were at the sicker end of the NYHA Class II-III spectrum.

Follow-up

As already stated, the average follow-up in the USCP was the shortest of the major beta-blocker mortality analyses (Appendix Table A3). This has implications for interpreting the risk reduction association with carvedilol; treatment effect is exaggerated by shorter follow-up. No patient was lost to mortality follow-up.

Haemodynamic effects

Heart rate decreased more in the carvedilol group (by 12.6 beats/minute) than in the placebo group (by 1.4 beats/minute, $p < 0.001$). Even though dizziness was a common complaint, mean blood pressure did not differ between the placebo and carvedilol groups.

Effects on primary endpoints of component trials in USCP

Though this review focuses on the mortality of the pooled USCP trials it should be pointed out that the component trials each had primary and secondary pre-specified endpoints.[11–14] These are listed in Table 9. The ability of the individuals trials to show a benefit of carvedilol was reduced by early termination of the US programme, such that recruitment and/or follow-up was incomplete in some of the component trials. In retrospect, it is also probable that exercise testing, a measure of treatment efficacy still in vogue at the time of the design of the USCP, was not a good endpoint to choose to measure the effect of a beta-blocker. Despite this, carvedilol improved the primary endpoint, progression of heart failure, in the "mild" trial (Figure 10).[11] One of the two primary exercise endpoints in the "moderate" PRECISE trial was also significantly improved. In addition, many of the secondary endpoints (Table 9) were improved by active therapy.[12]

Effects on mortality

Carvedilol reduced total mortality by 65% (95% CI 39–80), ie from 7.8% to 3.2% (31 of 398 placebo compared with 22 of 696 carvedilol patients), a highly significant effect (Figures 9 and 11, Appendix Table A5, $p < 0.001$).[4] This benefit of carvedilol was apparent across a large range of subgroups (Table 10). A new analysis has also shown mortality appears to be similarly reduced in blacks and non-blacks.[15] Superficially, the overall mortality effect of carvedilol seems much larger than that seen in either CIBIS-II,[6] in which there

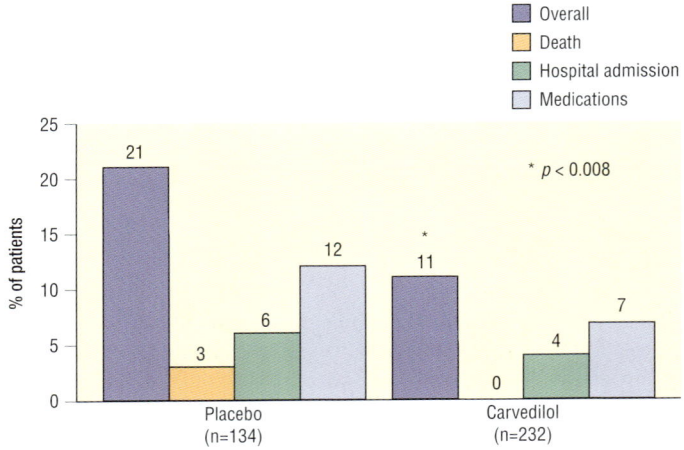

Figure 10
Effect of carvedilol on the clinical progression of CHF. Progression of CHF was defined as death due to CHF, hospitalization for CHF or the need to increase CHF medications.

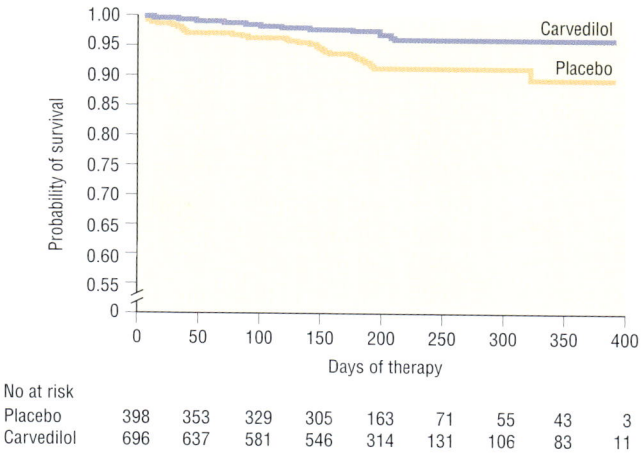

Figure 11
USCP survival curves.

was a 34% reduction (95% CI 19–46), or MERIT-HF,[7] in which the reduction was also 34% (95% CI 19–47). Of course, it is immediately apparent that the actual numbers were small: the mortality difference is based on nine deaths though the group sizes were different. The mortality relative risk reduction with carvedilol in the much sicker patients in COPERNICUS (which had an average follow-up of just under a year) was 35% (see page 52).

CIBIS-II and MERIT-HF were much larger studies (2647 and 3991 patients respectively, versus 1094 in USCP) and there were more deaths (384 and 362 in CIBIS-II and MERIT-HF, respectively, compared with 53 in the USCP trials). This means that the estimated risk reduction in CIBIS-II and MERIT-HF is much more robust and more likely to represent the "real" effect of beta-blockade in these patients. There are two other important issues to take into consideration when looking at the apparently large mortality risk reduction in the USCP. The first is the confounding effect of the open-label run-in period. At the time of termination of the USCP, 1197 patients had entered the open label run-in period. Of these, 5.6% had failed to complete the period because of adverse effects (including worsening heart failure in 1.4% and death in 0.6%). A further 3.0% failed to complete because of violations of the protocol or other administrative reasons. In CIBIS-II and MERIT-HF, patients not tolerating study drug, experiencing early adverse effects, not adhering to therapy or having events such as death or worsening heart failure counted in the intention-to-treat analysis from day 1 (since there was no pre-randomization run-in period to exclude such participants). It is difficult to know how to deal with this bias in favour of carvedilol. One way is to add all events occurring in the run-in period to the carvedilol group in the USCP.[16–18] Though this is a fairly harsh approach it does not substantially alter the overall conclusion from the USCP (the mortality risk reduction is a little less at 48% but still significant at $p = 0.011$).[17,18]

Another approach has been to do this "worst case" analysis and, in addition, pool the results of the USCP with those of another large carvedilol heart failure trial (the Australia–New Zealand trial),[5] the outline of which is shown in Figure 12. That trial did not show a reduction in mortality after a mean follow-up of 19 months (26 placebo versus 20 carvedilol deaths, relative risk 0.76, 95% CI 0.42–1.36, 2 $p = 0.1$).[5] This pooling gives an estimated relative risk of death with carvedilol, versus placebo, of 0.55 (95% CI 0.33–0.92), ie a 45% reduction in mortality with carvedilol.[19] However, this effect is achieved by adding a study with a difference of six deaths.

The second important issue affecting the interpretation of the size of the mortality reduction in the USCP is that of duration of follow-up. Short-term follow-up can exaggerate, and long-term follow-up diminish, the effect of therapy. Take, for example, the SOLVD treatment trial.[8] The mortality risk reduction at 3, 6 and 12 months was 33%, 29% and

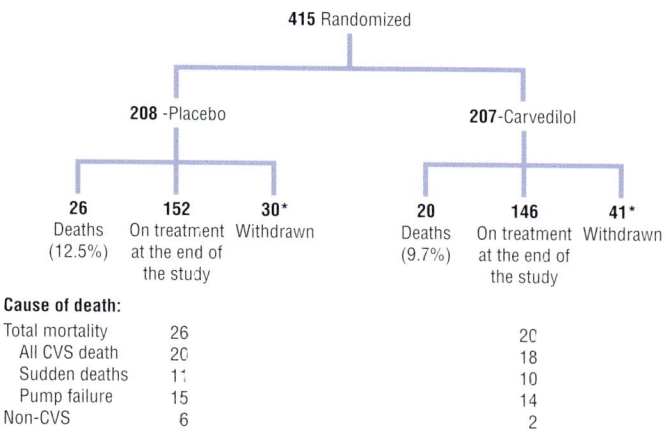

```
                        415 Randomized
                              |
        ┌─────────────────────┴─────────────────────┐
    208 -Placebo                                 207-Carvedilol
        |                                            |
  ┌─────┼─────┐                              ┌───────┼───────┐
 26      152    30*                         20       146     41*
Deaths On treatment Withdrawn             Deaths On treatment Withdrawn
(12.5%) at the end of                     (9.7%) at the end of
        the study                                the study
```

Cause of death:		
Total mortality	26	20
All CVS death	20	18
Sudden deaths	11	10
Pump failure	15	14
Non-CVS	6	2

* These figures have been derived by subtracting the numbers dying plus those still on treatment from the total number enrolled.

Figure 12
Australia and New Zealand carvedilol trial profile.

23% compared with 16% during the overall follow-up of 41.4 months. It is quite likely, therefore, that the short follow-up in the USCP has exaggerated the benefit of carvedilol; this is also generally true of all the beta-blocker trials (duration 0.5–1.3 years) compared with the landmark ACE inhibitor trial, SOLVD-T.[8]

Sudden death was reduced substantially in the USCP trials, as in the other trials, though this is based on 12 sudden deaths on carvedilol (of 696) and 15 in placebo (of 398, Appendix Table A5 and Figure 9). Also in keeping with the other trials, the mortality benefit from carvedilol was shown across a wide range of sub-groups

Effect of carvedilol on morbidity

Carvedilol reduced the proportion of patients requiring at least one hospital admission for a cardiovascular cause: 19.6% in the placebo group and 14.1% in the carvedilol group, a 27% (95% CI 3–45) risk reduction ($p = 0.036$).[4,15] The proportions admitted for any cause (27% versus 19%, relative risk 0.71, 95% CI 0.54–0.92) and for worsening CHF (9% versus 6%, relative risk 0.62, 95% CI 0.39–0.98) were also reduced significantly ($p = 0.009$ and 0.041, respectively, see Table 11). The combined endpoint of death or hospital admission for a cardiovascular reason was reduced from 24.6% in the placebo group to 15.8% in the carvedilol group, a 38% risk reduction (95% CI 18–53, $p < 0.001$). The same endpoint was reduced from 35 to 29% in CIBIS-II, a risk reduction of 21% (95% CI 10–31, $p = 0.0004$). The total number of hospital admissions (any cause) in the placebo group was 160 (0.40 ± SD 0.78 per patient) and 208 (0.30 ± 0.78 per patient) in the carvedilol group ($p = 0.003$). The numbers of cardiovascular (119 versus 143, $p = 0.021$) and CHF (61 versus 52, $p = 0.028$) hospital admissions were also reduced with carvedilol (Table 11).

A new analysis has shown that carvedilol seems to reduce morbidity and improve symptoms in patients with atrial fibrillation as well as those in sinus rhythm.[20]

By reducing hospital admissions, carvedilol was cost-effective in the USCP.[21]

Dosing

The target dose of carvedilol in the USCP was 25 mg twice daily (50 mg bid in patients ≥85 kg). A very high percentage of patients appeared to reach target dose in the USCP trials, though it must be remembered that this proportion will have been inflated by exclusion of intolerant patients during the open-label run-in period (Appendix Table A6).[4]

Tolerability and adverse effects

The main results paper of the USCP[4] only describes permanent discontinuations because of adverse reactions (cf main reports of CIBIS-II and MERIT-HF, which describe overall discontinuation rates).[4,6,7] 7.8% of the placebo group and 5.7% of the carvedilol group in the USCP stopped treatment because of adverse reactions (a subsequent MERIT-HF report gives equivalent placebo and metoprolol CR/XL rates of 11.7% and 9.8%).[22] Analysis of the reports of the individual component trials of the USCP,[11–14] however, gives overall discontinuation rates of 18.3% in the placebo group and 10.8% in the carvedilol group, proportions very similar to CIBIS-II (15% in both treatment groups) and MERIT-HF (15.3% in the placebo group and 13.9% in the metoprolol group). It is very difficult, however, to compare adverse event rates and discontinuation rates in the USCP with the other trials because of the exclusion of patients intolerant of carvedilol during the open-label run-in phase.

With this caveat in mind, the overall rates of adverse reactions in the USCP are shown in Appendix Table A7, which also shows the rates reported for CIBIS-II (these data are not available for MERIT-HF). The rates are broadly similar, with the exception of dizziness, which seems to be more common with carvedilol, possibly because of its alpha-adrenoceptor antagonist action. Even if real, however, this excess of dizziness did not seem to result in more discontinuation of double-blind therapy (see below and Appendix Table A7).

The main report of the USCP mortality analysis and the reports of the individual component trials give a great deal more interesting information on adverse events.[4,11–14] These data detail adverse events during initiation, up-titration and maintenance, allow comparison between adverse event rates in patients with milder CHF and in those with more severe CHF, and allow comparison of lower and higher dose carvedilol treatment. A thorough review of these data is beyond the scope of this chapter, although some general points can be made. Dizziness seemed to be the most common adverse event reported during treatment initiation (in around 13–15% of patients in the open-label challenge phase). Worsening CHF appeared to occur a bit more commonly in more severe cases (7.3% in moderately severe versus 4.0% in mild) during the open-label challenge phase, and carvedilol withdrawals were more common in patients with more severe CHF during this phase (8.0% versus 5.9%). Worsening heart failure was a bit more common in the carvedilol group than in the placebo group during the up-titration phase, but this effect was reversed during maintenance therapy (ie worsening CHF was more common in the placebo group during this later phase).

The unique design of the USCP, in having an open-label run-in period, also allows comparison between the adverse events related to initiation of an ACE inhibitor and a beta-blocker. The SOLVD trials also had an open-label enalapril run-in period.[8] The median duration of the open-label challenge in the SOLVD trials was 7 days and 98/7487 (1.3%) of patients had to stop treatment because of an adverse effect (2.6% of NYHA Class III/IV patients). The duration of the open-label phase of the USCP was 14 days and 67 (5.6%) of 1197 patients had to stop treatment. 15% of patients with mild CHF and 13.6% of patients with moderately severe CHF reported dizziness in the USCP compared with 6.4% in SOLVD-T. Adverse effects from carvedilol are, therefore, probably a bit more common than with an ACE inhibitor.

The most common specific adverse events *leading to discontinuation of double-blind therapy* are also described and can be compared to MERIT-HF (Appendix Table A7).[22] All such events were infrequent and only a small excess of bradycardia and dizziness was reported in the carvedilol group. Dizziness and hypotension did not seem to be more frequent in the USCP than in MERIT-HF though the latter had a longer follow-up and the former introduced a bias by having an open-label run-in phase that will have selected patients able to tolerate carvedilol.

The COPERNICUS trial

The primary objective of COPERNICUS was to examine the effect of carvedilol, added to conventional therapy, on all-cause mortality in patients with *severe* symptomatic chronic heart failure caused by reduced left ventricular systolic function. COPERNICUS was a large, randomized, multicentre trial (sites in 14 European countries, Israel, South Africa, USA, Canada, Australia, Argentina and Mexico).[23]

A total of 2289 patients were enrolled; the inclusion criteria are set out in Appendix Table A3. All patients had an ejection fraction of less than 0.25, a much lower figure than in the other big beta-blocker trials. Unlike the other trials, the aim was to recruit high-risk patients and as a consequence, patients were required to have "symptoms of dyspnoea and/or fatigue at rest or on minimal exertion for at least 2 months". The main exclusion criteria were: use of intravenous positive inotropic or vasodilator agents (except digitalis) within 4 days of the screening phase (the time between screening and randomization was 3–14 days), a systolic blood pressure of less than 85 mm Hg and a serum creatinine of more than 247.5 µmol/l (and no increase of more than 44.2 µmol/l during screening). Diuretic therapy should have been optimized before randomization with no or minimal oedema present.

Carvedilol was started at a dose of 3.125 mg twice daily and increased at intervals of at least 2 weeks to 6.25 mg, 12.5 mg and 25 mg twice daily, if tolerated.

Results

The study was stopped prematurely on the recommendation of the independent safety committee. The mean follow-up time was 10.4 months. The trial profile is presented in Figure 13. 130 patients on carvedilol and 190 on placebo died (p = 0.0014). The mortality rates were 11.4% and 18.5% per patient year of follow-up with a hazard ratio of 0.65 (95% CI 0.52–0.81, Figure 14).

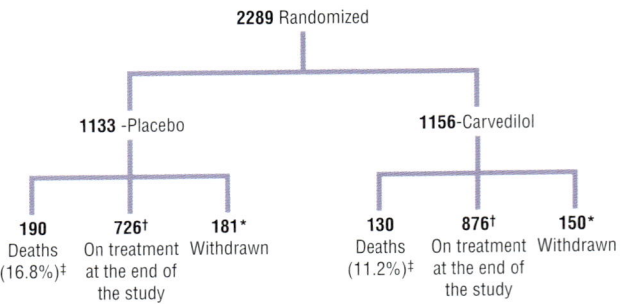

*Figures calculated from reported 16% placebo and 13% carvedilol premature discontinuation of therapy rates; †This figure derived by subtracting those dying and withdrawn from total number randomized; ‡Figure not annualized.

Figure 13
COPERNICUS trial profile.

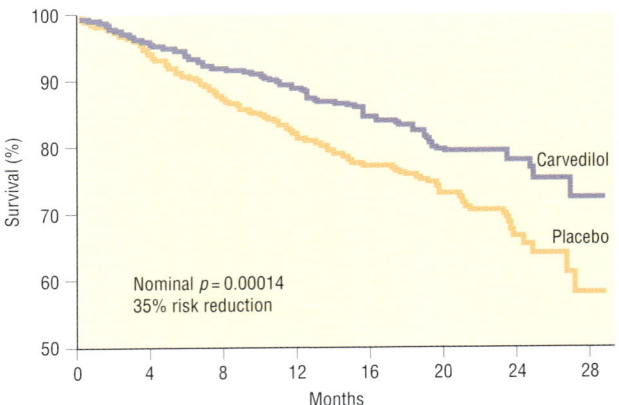

Figure 14
Copernicus survival curves.

Detailed evaluation of the COPERNICUS trial

In this section the design and results of COPERNICUS are compared with the USCP, CIBIS-II and MERIT-HF. The details of the design, conduct and inclusion criteria of the three trials are presented in Appendix Tables A1 and A2. The characteristics of the patients enrolled are set out in Appendix Table A3. These are provisional as the trial has yet to be published in full.

Entry criteria

The enrolment criteria were very different to those in the other trials, as outlined earlier. The objective was to recruit many more symptomatic and higher risk patients.

Details of patients

The patients enrolled in COPERNICUS were similar in age to those in MERIT-HF and CIBIS-II and older than patients in the USCP. All patients were, by definition, in NYHA Class III and IV and, per protocol, had a much lower mean LVEF (0.20) than any of the other trials (0.23 in USCP, 0.28 in CIBIS-II, and 0.28 in MERIT-HF). Patients in COPERNICUS had a surprisingly well maintained systolic blood pressure (123 mm Hg) and no more tachycardia than in the other trials (the entry heart rate could not be < 68 beats/minute).

Event rates

In keeping with the trial objectives, greater severity of symptoms and lower LVEF, COPERNICUS patients had the highest mortality of all the big beta-blocker trials. The placebo group's annualized mortality was 18.5%. The mortality rates in NYHA Class III and IV patients in CIBIS-II[6] were 15.8 and 24.6%, respectively, and in MERIT-HF[7] were 13.2% and 24.9%, respectively, very much in keeping with COPERNICUS. However, other recent trials, recruiting CHF patients with severe symptoms, reported higher mortality rates. For example, the 1-year mortality rate in the placeholder group of RALES was roughly 25%.[24] Other placebo-group mortality rates include 24% in PROMISE (after a mean follow-up of 6.1 months),[25] 38% in PRAISE (13.8 months),[26] 20% in PRIME-2 (12 months),[27] and 19% in the vesnarinone study (9 months).[28] Consequently, it is clear that even COPERNICUS did not recruit the most severely ill patients with CHF, eg the most elderly, oedematous, patients admitted to hospital and those requiring current intravenous therapy.

Follow-up

The mean follow-up in COPERNICUS (10.4 months) was slightly shorter than in CIBIS-II (1.3 years) and MERIT-HF (1.0 years, Appendix Table A3).

Effects on mortality

Carvedilol reduced total mortality by 35% (hazard ratio 0.65, 95% CI 0.52–0.81), an almost identical effect to that of bisoprolol in CIBIS-II and metoprolol CR/XL in MERIT-HF (Figure 14). This mortality benefit was shown across a wide range of patient sub-groups (Figure 15). Interesting *post hoc* but blinded, sub-group analyses were also done to examine the most severely ill patients randomized in COPERNICUS. The following describes the provisional findings in these analyses. One sub-group was those patients with a LVEF of less than 0.20 and a hospital admission for CHF in the past year. 22 (17.9%) of 191 carvedilol-treated patients died, compared with 36 (22.5%) of 188 patients on placebo, giving a hazard ratio of 0.58 (95% CI 0.34–0.98). The second high-risk sub-group included patients with a LVEF of less than 0.15 and more than three hospital admissions with worsening heart failure in the year before randomization. 39 (19%) of 246 patients treated with carvedilol died, compared with 61 (25%) of 265 placebo-treated patients, giving a hazard ratio of 0.64 (95% CI 0.43–0.96). Lastly, a sub-group was identified of patients admitted to hospital at entry, with evidence of sodium and water retention, who had received

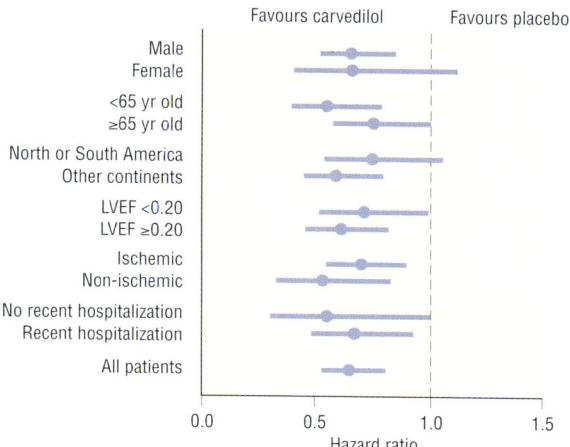

Figure 15

Hazard ratios (and 95 per cent confidence intervals) for death from any cause in subgroups defined according to base-line characteristics.
LVEF denotes left ventricle ejection fraction. Recent hospitalization refers to hospitalization for heart failure within the year before enrolment. Reproduced with permission from Packer.[23]

recent intravenous vasodilator or positive inotropic therapy or had been admitted to hospital more than three times with worsening heart failure in the past year. The mortality rate in patients given carvedilol was 16.7% (16/151), compared with 25.3% (32/153) in the placebo group, giving a hazard ratio of 0.50 (95% CI 0.25–0.90).

A new analysis of MERIT-HF, involving post-hoc selection of 'COPERNICUS-like' patients has shown similar event reductions with metoprolol.[29] A similar analysis has been carried out for CIBIS-II.[30]

Effects on morbidity

The effect of carvedilol on composite morbidity mortality end-points has been described. The following reductions have been reported: 24% death or hospitalization for any cause (Figure 16, $p < 0.001$), 27% death or hospitalization for a cardiovascular reason ($p < 0.0001$) and 31% for death or hospitalization for heart failure ($p < 0.0001$). A total of 507 patients in the placebo group and 425 in the carvedilol group died or were hospitalized.

Dosing

The target dose of carvedilol in COPERNICUS was 25 mg twice daily. 65.1% of patients were titrated at some point in the first 4 months of the trial, to the target dose (the equivalent rate in the placebo group was 78.2%). The mean daily doses of placebo and carvedilol were 41 mg and 37 mg respectively. These are remarkably good figures, especially since there was no open-label run-in phase, as in the USCP. The proportion of patients reaching the target dose of therapy in CIBIS-II was 43% and in MERIT-HF 64% (Appendix Table A7).

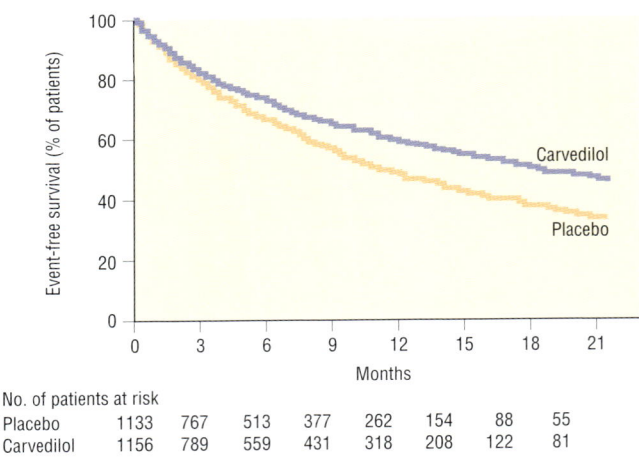

No. of patients at risk								
Placebo	1133	767	513	377	262	154	88	55
Carvedilol	1156	789	559	431	318	208	122	81

Figure 16
Kaplan–Meier analysis of time to death or first hospitalization for any reason in the placebo group and the carvedilol group.
The 24 per cent lower risk in the carvedilol group was significant (P<0.001).
Reproduced with permission from Packer et al.[23]

Tolerability and adverse effects

In COPERNICUS, 14.8% of carvedilol-treated and 18.5% of placebo-treated patients were withdrawn from randomized therapy within 12 months. The permanent discontinuation rate in CIBIS-II was 15% in both groups, and was 13.9% of the metoprolol group and 15.3% of the placebo group in MERIT-HF.

References

1. Frishman WH . Carvedilol. *N Engl J Med* 1998; **339:** 1759–65.
2. Yue T-L, Cheng H-Y, Lysko PG, et al. Carvedilol, a new vasodilator and beta adrenoceptor antagonist, is an antioxidant and free radical scavenger. *J Pharmacol Exper Therapeut* 1992; **263:** 92–8.
3. Kukin ML, Kalman J, Charney RH, et al. Prospective, randomised comparison of effect of long-term treatment with metoprolol or carvedilol on symptoms, exercise, ejection fraction, and oxidative stress in heart failure. *Circulation* 1999; **99:** 2645–51.
4. Packer M, Bristow MR, Cohn JN, et al, and the US Carvedilol Heart Failure Study Group. The effect of carvedilol on morbidity and mortality in patients with chronic heart failure. *N Engl J Med* 1996; **334:** 1349–55.
5. Australia/New Zealand Heart Failure Research Collaborative Group. Randomised, placebo-controlled trial of carvedilol in patients with congestive heart failure due to ischaemic heart disease. *Lancet* 1997; **349:** 375–80.
6. CIBIS-II Investigators and Committees. The cardiac insufficiency bisoprolol study II (CIBIS-II) a randomised trial. *Lancet* 1999; **353:** 9–13.
7. MERIT-HF Study Group. Effect of metoprolol CR/XL in chronic heart failure: metoprolol CR/XL randomised intervention trial in congestive heart failure (MERIT-HF). *Lancet* 1999; **353:** 2001–7.
8. Yusuf S. Effect of enalapril on survival in patients with reduced left ventricular ejection fractions and congestive heart failure. *N Engl J Med* 1991; **325**(5): 293–302.
9. Poole Wilson P, Cleland J, Hubbard W, et al. Clinical outcome with enalapril in symptomatic chronic heart failure: a dose comparison. *Eur Heart J* 1998; **19**(3): 481–9.
10. Pitt B, Segal R, Martinez FA et al, and the ELITE study investigators. Randomised trial of losartan versus captopril in patients over 65 with heart failure (Evaluation of losartan in the elderly study, ELITE). *Lancet* 1997; **349:** 747–52.
11. Colucci WS, Packer M, Bristow MR, Gilbert EM, Cohn JN. Carvedilol inhibits clinical progression in patients with mild symptoms of heart failure. *Circulation* 1996; **94:** 2800–6.

12. Packer M, Colucci WS, Sackner-Bernstein JD, Liang CS. Double-blind, placebo-controlled study of the effects of carvedilol in patients with moderate to severe heart failure – the PRECISE trial. *Circulation* 1996; **94**(11): 2793–9.

13. Bristow MR, Gilbert EM, Abraham WT. Carvedilol produces dose-related improvements in left ventricular function and survival in sujects with chronic heart failure. *Circulation* 1996; **94**: 2807–16.

14. Cohn JN. Safety and efficacy of carvedilol in severe heart failure. The US Carvedilol Heart Failure Study Group. *J Cardiol Fail* 1997; **3**(3): 173–9.

15. Yancy CW, Fowler MB, Colucci WS, et al of the U.S. Carvedilol Heart Failure Study Group. Race and the response to adrenergic blockade with carvedilol in patients with chronic heart failure. *N Engl J Med* 2001; **344**: 1358–65.

16. Von Olshausen K, Pop T, Berger J. Carvedilol in patients with chronic heart failure. *N Engl J Med* 1996; **335**: 1318–19.

17. Packer M, Cohn JN, Colucci WS. Carvedilol in patients with chronic heart failure – reply. *N Engl J Med* 1996; **335**:1319–20.

18. Packer M. Effects of beta-adrenergic blockade on survival of patients with chronic heart failure. *Am J Cardiol* 1997; **80**: L46–L54.

19. Schmidt BMW, Janson CP, Wehling M. Assuming the worst may not be bad at all – carvedilol in heart failure treatment. *Eur J Clin Pharmacol* 1998; **54**(4): 282–5.

20. Joglar JA, Acusta AP, Shusterman NH, et al. Effect of carvedilol on survival and hemodynamics in patients with atrial fibrillation and left ventricle dysfunction: retrospective analysis of the US Carvedilol Heart Failure Trials Program. *Am Heart J* 2001; **142**: 498–501.

21. Fowler MB, Vera-Llonch M, Oster G, et al. Influence of carvedilol on hospitalizations in heart failure: incidence, resource utilization and costs. U.S. Carvedilol Heart Failure Study Group. *J Am Coll Cardiol* 2001; **37**: 1692–9.

22. Hjalmarson A, Goldstein S, Fagerberg B, et al. Effects of controlled-release metoprolol on total mortality, hospitalizations, and well-being in patients with heart failure: the Metoprolol CR/XL Randomized Intervention Trial in congestive heart failure (MERIT-HF). MERIT-HF Study Group. *JAMA* 2000; **283**: 1295–302.

23. Packer M, Coats AJ, Fowler MB, et al for the Carvedilol Prospective Randomized Cumulative Survival Study Group. Effect of carvedilol on survival in severe chronic heart failure. *N Engl J Med* 2001; **344**: 1651–8.

24. Pitt B, Zannad F, Remme WJ, and the Randomized Aldactone evaluation study investigators. The effect of spironolactone on morbidity and mortality in patients with severe heart failure. *N Engl J Med* 1999; **341**: 709–17.

25. Packer M, Carver JR, Rodeheffer RJ. Effect of oral milrinone on mortality in severe chronic heart failure. *N Engl J Med* 1991; **325**(21): 1468–75.

26. O'Connor CM, Carson PE, Miller AB, et al, and the PRAISE Investigators. Effect of amlodipine on mode of death among patients with advanced heart failure in the PRAISE trial. *Am J Cardiol* 1998; **82:** 881–7.

27. Hampton JR, Van Veldhuisen DJ, Cowley AJ, Kleber FX, Charlesworth A. Achieving appropriate endpoints in heart failure trials: the PRIME-II protocol. *Eur J Heart Failure* 1999; **1:** 89–93.

28. Cohn JN, Goldstein SO, Greenberg BH, et al. A dose-dependent increase in mortality with vesnarinone among patients with severe heart failure. *N Engl J Med* 1998; **339:** 1810–16.

29. Goldstein S, Fagerberg B, Hjalmarson A, et al. Metoprolol controlled release/extended release in patients with severe heart failure. Analysis of the experience in the MERIT-HF study. *J Am Coll Cardiol* 2001; **38:** 932–8.

30. Erdmann E, Lechat P, Verkenne P, Wiemann H. Results from post-hoc analyses of the CIBIS II trial: effect of bisoprolol in high-risk patient groups with chronic heart failure. *Eur J Heart Fail* 2001; **3:** 469–79

Bisoprolol is a beta$_1$ selective adrenoceptor antagonist with neither intrinsic sympathomimetic nor membrane stabilizing activity, 50% is metabolized by the liver, 50% is excreted unchanged by the kidney. The half-life is 10–12 hours. It was originally licensed for the treatment of hypertension and angina at a dose of 5 or 10 mg once daily. Its role in heart failure has been demonstrated by two trials: CIBIS,[1] now sometimes called CIBIS-I; and more importantly by CIBIS-II.[2] Only the latter was powered to show a significant effect on mortality. CIBIS-II is the subject of this chapter, and brief mention is made of the first CIBIS study since it had an effect on the design of CIBIS-II.

CIBIS-I

CIBIS (Cardiac Insufficiency Bisoprolol Study) was the first large-scale placebo controlled study to assess the effect of a beta$_1$ selective beta-blocker on mortality rates in patients with heart failure. They were all receiving standard therapy with diuretics and a vasodilator, usually an ACE inhibitor. In total, 641 patients with CHF due to a variety of causes, and belonging to NYHA classes III (95%) or IV and having an ejection fraction of less than 40% were included. The initial dose of bisoprolol was 1.25 mg daily and the aim was to titrate the dose up to 5 mg daily. One month after the last increment a mean heart-rate reduction of 15.7 beats per minute had been achieved. At that time the mean daily dose was 4.5 mg on placebo and 3.8 mg on bisoprolol. 59% of patients had reached the target dose of 5 mg daily.

The 2-year mortality rates did not differ significantly between bisoprolol (53/320, 16.6%) and placebo (67/321, 20.9%), although mortality on bisoprolol was 20% lower than on placebo. The study was underpowered, the population of patients studied was too small and the placebo annual mortality rate of 11.2% was lower than expected. However, bisoprolol did improve the functional status and did seem to have a more marked effect on those patients with a "non-ischaemic cardiomyopathy".

On the basis of the information obtained, CIBIS-II was designed. Subsequently, studies on patients in CIBIS-I showed that the improvement in left ventricular function noted in those studied correlated well with heart-rate reduction.[3] This effect was attributable in part to increased vagal tone. Bisoprolol also increased left ventricular fractional shortening and this was associated with decreased risk of deaths or with improved survival rates.[3]

CIBIS-II

CIBIS-II was a multicentre randomized placebo-controlled trial of patients aged 18–80 years with an ejection fraction of 35% or less. The patients were recruited in Europe and details of the trial are given in Appendix Tables A1–A7. The primary aim was to assess the effect of bisoprolol added to conventional therapy on all-cause mortality in patients with moderate to severe heart failure caused by reduced left ventricular systolic function. Patients had to have typical heart failure symptoms and to be in NYHA III or IV and be stabilized on diuretics and an ACE inhibitor (or an alternative vasodilator). In addition to various cardiac exclusion criteria, resting heart rate had to be 60 or more beats per minute, systolic pressure above 100 mmHg and serum creatinine less than 300 μmol/l. Patients with cardiac failure of different types were grouped into three categories: ischaemic heart disease based on angiography or a proven myocardial infarct; dilated cardiomyopathy with normal coronary arteries; and others, which included hypertension, valvular disease and suspected but unproven ischaemic heart disease.

Bisoprolol was started at a dose of 1.25 mg daily and increased at weekly intervals and subsequently at 4-weekly intervals through 2.5, 3.75, 5, and 7.5 to 10 mg daily.

The primary endpoint was all-cause mortality. Secondary endpoints were all-cause hospital admissions, cardiovascular mortality and cardiovascular hospital admissions and permanent premature treatment withdrawals.

Results

2647 patients were randomized and followed for a mean of 1.3 years. Baseline characteristics in the two groups were similar. The trial format and the key results are presented in Figure 17. The trial was stopped prematurely because the efficacy of bisoprolol had been demonstrated, 156 versus 228 deaths ($p < 0.0001$). The estimated annual mortality rates were 8.8% in the bisoprolol group and 13.2% in the placebo group (hazard ratio 0.66, 95%CI 0.54–0.81).

Bisoprolol reduced sudden deaths by 44%. The effect on mortality was similar in those with ischaemic and those with non-ischaemic heart failure, those with NYHA class III and those in class IV. Admissions to hospital were also reduced, with admissions for heart failure reduced by 32% ($p < 0.0001$). There were, however, more admissions for

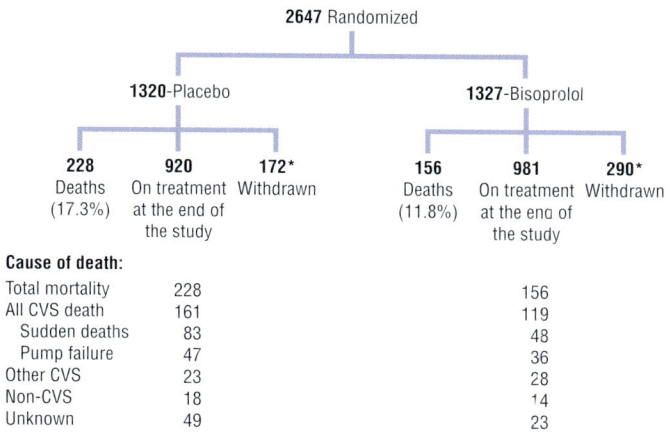

2647 Randomized

1320-Placebo | **1327**-Bisoprolol

	Placebo			Bisoprolol	
228 Deaths (17.3%)	**920** On treatment at the end of the study	**172*** Withdrawn	**156** Deaths (11.8%)	**981** On treatment at the end of the study	**290*** Withdrawn

Cause of death:

Total mortality	228	156
All CVS death	161	119
Sudden deaths	83	48
Pump failure	47	36
Other CVS	23	28
Non-CVS	18	14
Unknown	49	23

*These figures were derived by subtracting the numbers dying plus those still on treatment from the total number entered.

Figure 17
CIBIS-II Trial profile.

stroke (31 versus 16, $p = 0.04$). 564 patients reached the target dose of 10 mg daily, 152 reached 7.5 mg and 176 reached 5 mg.

Detailed evaluation of CIBIS-II

In this section, the design and results of CIBIS-II are compared with MERIT-HF,[4] the US Carvedilol Programme (USCP),[5] and the COPERNICUS trial, details of which are given in the other chapters. The details of the design, conduct and the inclusion criteria of the four trials are presented in Appendix Tables A1 and A2. The characteristics of the patients enrolled, endpoints and annual mortality rates for the three trials are set out in Appendix Table A3 and the concomitant medication in Appendix Table A4.

The entry criteria should have resulted in CIBIS-II[2] having a higher mortality and morbidity rate than the USCP and MERIT-HF trials. MERIT-HF and the USCP recruited patients with NYHA class II–IV CHF whereas CIBIS-II sought Class III and IV patients only. COPERNICUS also intended to recruit NYHA Class III and IV patients, with a lower LVEF. Patients entering CIBIS-II could be treated with amiodarone, whereas concomitant treatment with this antiarrhythmic agent was excluded by the other trials.[2,4,5]

Event rates

There were seven times as many deaths in CIBIS–II as in the USCP; Figure 17, Appendix Tables A3 and A5).[2] The annual mortality rate of 13.2% (17.3% over the whole follow-up period) was a little higher than in MERIT-HF though similar to that in NYHA Class III and IV patients in MERIT-HF. The placebo group mortality rates in Class III and IV patients were 15.8% and 24.6% in CIBIS-II and 13.2% and 24.9% in MERIT-HF; the average follow-up was, however, longer in CIBIS-II than MERIT-HF (see below). The patients enrolled in the placebo group of COPERNICUS (18.5%) had a much higher annualized mortality than CIBIS-II (13.2%). The CIBIS–II mortality rate was also lower than in other recent trials recruiting Class III and IV patients. Placebo group mortality in PROMISE was 24% after a mean follow-up of 6.1 months, in PRAISE 38% (over 13.8 months), in PRIME-2 20% (over 12 months), and 19% (over 9 months) in the vesnarinone CHF mortality study.[6–9] By contrast, the 1-year mortality rate in SOLVD-T (57% NYHA class II) was 12.3%.[10] The proportion of patients dying suddenly seemed to be much smaller in CIBIS-II than MERIT-HF (Appendix Table A5). This may reflect a different endpoint classification system and/or the high proportion of patients with more severe CHF who are more likely to die from pump failure than suddenly.[4]

The main CIBIS-II results paper gives much more information on morbidity than either of the other two trial main reports,[2] though a detailed supplementary MERIT-HF paper describing morbidity has been published[11] (at the time of writing, COPERNICUS has not been published). In CIBIS-II the proportion of patients admitted to hospital in the placebo group (diuretic, ACE inhibitor and/or digoxin) was 39% for any cause and 18% for worsening CHF; the proportion dying or being admitted to hospital for a cardio-vascular reason was 35%. These rates also seem a little low for true NYHA Class III/IV patients. In the PRIME-2 study the proportion of patients in the placebo group admit-ted to hospital during a mean follow-up of 1-year was 44%.[8] In the vesnarinone CHF mortality study, the propor-tion of patients admitted to hospital for worsening CHF during a mean follow-up of 9 months was 18.5%; in that study the proportion dying or requiring hospital admission for CHF was 29.8%.[9] In the DIG trial (in which 54% of patients were NYHA class II) the 1-year rate of death or hospital admission for any reason was 41% in the digoxin group; the rate for cardiovascular death or cardiovascular hospital admission was 32%.[12]

MERIT-HF does not report exactly the same morbidity end-points as CIBIS-II. However, 38% of placebo-group patients died or were admitted to hospital for any reason in this trial. 33% of placebo-treated patients were admitted to hospital at least once (for any reason) and 14.7% for wors-ening CHF. These rates are a little lower than in CIBIS-II, in keeping with the broader entry criteria.

Follow-up

The average follow-up in CIBIS-II (1.3 years) was the longest of the major beta-blocker trials (with the exception of BEST). Six patients (five in the bisoprolol group) were lost to follow-up.[2]

Haemodynamic effects

No haemodynamic effects are reported in the main results paper from CIBIS-II.[2]

Effect on mortality

Bisoprolol reduced total mortality by 34% (Figures 17 and 18).[2] The total number of deaths was 228 (17.3%) in the placebo group and 156 (11.8%) in the bisoprolol group ($p < 0.0001$). The estimated annual mortality rate was 13.2% in the placebo group and 8.8% in the bisoprolol group (hazard ratio 0.66, 95% CI 0.54–0.81). Sudden death was reduced by 44% in the bisoprolol group (Appendix Table A5 and Figure 17). This mortality benefit was seen across a wide range of sub-groups in CIBIS-II (Figure 19). These findings are very similar to MERIT-HF, in which all-cause mortality was reduced by 34% from 11.0% to 7.2% per patient year of follow up. Sudden death was reduced by 41% in MERIT-HF (see next chapter). New extensive, post hoc sub-group analyses examining high-risk groups (e.g. NYHA Class IV), co-morbidity (e.g. diabetes mellitus) and concomitant therapy (e.g. spironolactone) have also been published, showing consistent benefit of bisoprolol.[13] Another recent post hoc sub-group

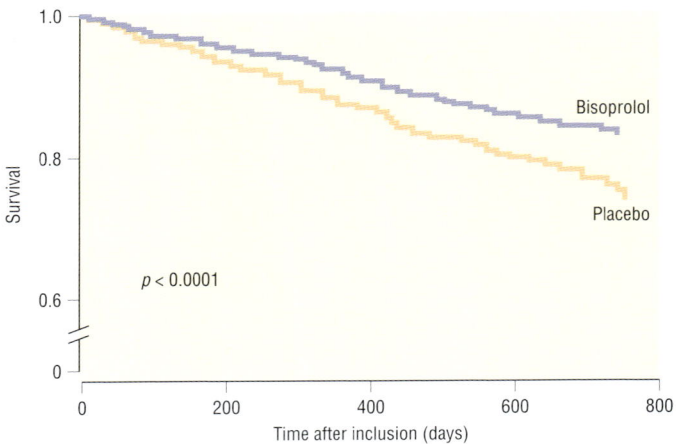

Figure 18
CIBIS-II survival curves.

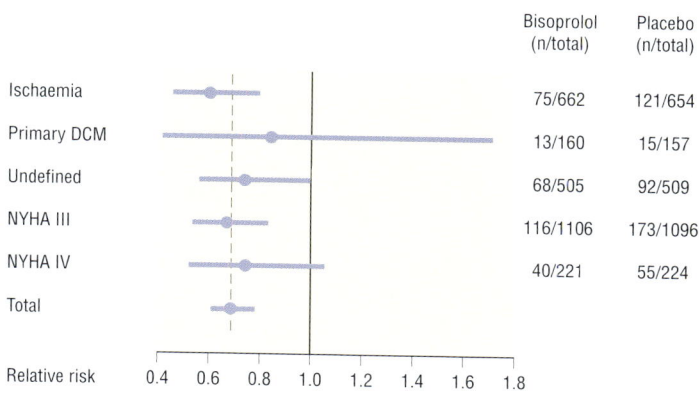

	Bisoprolol (n/total)	Placebo (n/total)
Ischaemia	75/662	121/654
Primary DCM	13/160	15/157
Undefined	68/505	92/509
NYHA III	116/1106	173/1096
NYHA IV	40/221	55/224
Total		

Relative risk   0.4   0.6   0.8   1.0   1.2   1.4   1.6   1.8

Figure 19

Relative risk of treatment effect on mortality by aetiology and functional class at baseline. Horizontal bars represent 95% CI.

analysis has, however, suggested that bisoprolol may not reduce mortality in patients with atrial fibrillation.[14]

Effect of bisoprolol on morbidity

Bisoprolol had a striking effect on cardiovascular morbidity as well as mortality.[2] Significantly fewer bisoprolol patients (33%) than placebo patients (39%) required a hospital admission (Figure 20, hazard ratio 0.80, 95% CI 0.71–0.91, $p = 0.0006$). This is similar to the effect of carvedilol in the USCP (19% versus 27%, RR 0.71, 95% CI 0.54–0.92, $p = 0.009$) and metoprolol in MERIT-HF (29.1% versus 33.3%, relative risk reduction, RRR 13%, $p = 0.004$). Hospital admission for heart failure was also significantly less common in the bisoprolol group (12% of patients) than in the placebo group (18%) hazard ratio 0.64, (95% CI 0.53–0.79, $p = 0.0001$). This is also similar to the USCP (6% versus 9%, RR 0.62, 95% CI 0.39–0.98, $p = 0.041$) and MERIT-HF (10% versus 14.7%, RRR 32%, $p < 0.001$). There were also fewer hospital admissions in

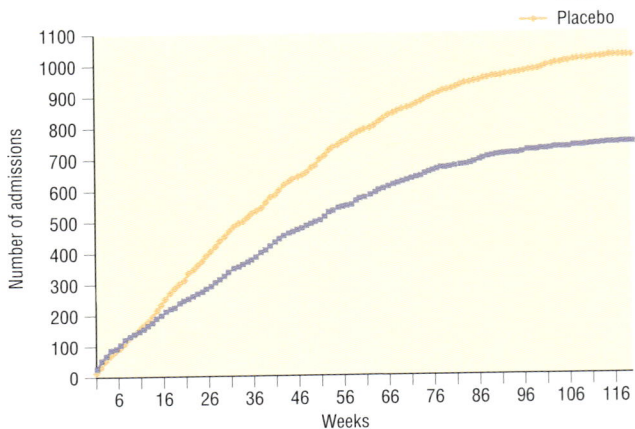

Figure 20
Cumulative number of hospital admissions in CIBIS-II.

the bisoprolol group for ventricular arrhythmias (six versus 20, $p=0.006$) and hypotension (three versus 11, $p=0.03$). There were, however, more admissions in the bisoprolol group for stroke (31 versus 16, $p=0.04$) and bradycardia (14 versus two, $p < 0.004$). There was no difference between the groups for other types of hospital admission.

Dosing

The proportion of patients (43%) reaching target dose (10 mg), or half target dose, was lower in CIBIS-II than in the USCP or MERIT-HF studies (Appendix Table A6). Why this should be is not clear. One possibility, however, is that CIBIS-II recruited sicker patients (more NYHA Class III and IV) than in these other two trials and these patients may have been less able to tolerate larger beta-blocker doses (see USCP adverse events, above). The proportion reaching target dose in the USCP will have been exaggerated by the programmed design (open-label run-in, see above). Even so, the proportion of patients reaching target dose in CIBIS-II is still lower than in MERIT-HF (64%) and COPERNICUS (65.1%), though the target dose of carvedilol in COPERNICUS was lower than in the USCP. In COPERNICUS the 65.1% of patients achieved the target dose of 25 mg bd at some stage in the first 4 months of the trial (see previous chapter).

Tolerability and adverse effects

The proportion of patients discontinuing study drug was the same on the placebo and active therapy groups (15%) and was similar to that in MERIT-HF (13.9% in the metoprolol group) and COPERNICUS (14.8% in the carvedilol group).[2] The placebo-corrected rates of adverse events in CIBIS-II were very similar to those reported in the USCP trials with the exception of dizziness (3% excess in CIBIS-II, 13% excess in the USCP; Appendix Table A7). As mentioned earlier, this difference may reflect the alpha-blocking action of carvedilol. Overall adverse event rates are not available for MERIT-HF.

Economic analysis of CIBIS-II

An economic analysis of CIBIS-II has been done for the UK, France and Germany. This analysis shows that the overall cost of care was less with adjunctive bisoprolol treatment than with placebo in all three countries studied (Figure 21).[15] This conclusion was reached even though the cost of extra hospital/office visits was added for the initiation and up-titration of bisoprolol therapy. This finding makes beta-blockers all the more remarkable a treatment for CHF.

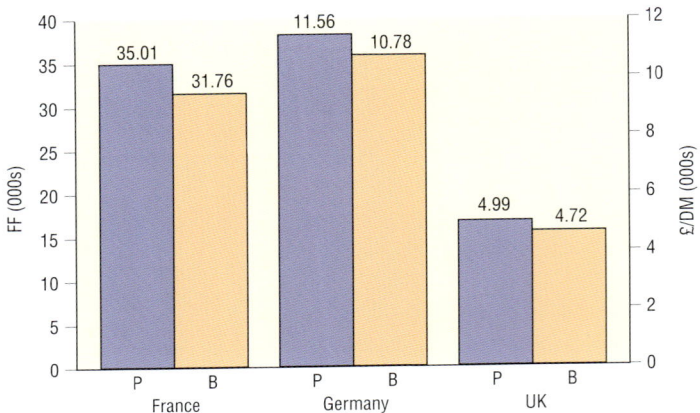

Figure 21
Total cost per patient treated in CIBIS-II; P = placebo; B = bisoprolol.

References

1. CIBIS Investigators and Committees. A randomized trial of beta-blockade in heart failure. *Circulation* 1994; **90:** 1765–73.
2. CIBIS-II Investigators and Committees. The cardiac insufficiency Bisoprolol Study II (CIBIS-II) a randomised trial. *Lancet* 1999; **353:** 9–13.
3. Lechat P, Escolano S, Golmard JL, et al. Prognostic value of bisoprolol induced hemodynamic effects in heart failure during the Cardiac Insufficiency Bisoprolol Study (CIBIS). *Circulation* 1997; **96:** 2197–205.
4. MERIT-HF Study Group. Effect of metoprolol CR/XL in chronic heart failure: metoprolol CR/XL randomised intervention trial in congestive heart failure (MERIT-HF). *Lancet* 1999; **353:** 2001–7.
5. Packer M, Bristow MR, Cohn JN, et al, and the US Carvedilol Heart Failure Study Group. The effect of carvedilol on morbidity and mortality in patients with chronic heart failure. *N Engl J Med* 1996; **334:** 1349–55.
6. Packer M, Carver JR, Rodeheffer RJ. Effect of oral milrinone on mortality in severe chronic heart failure. *N Engl J Med* 1991; **325:** 1468–75.
7. Packer M, O'Connor C, Ghali J, et al, and the Prospective Randomized Amlodipine Survival Evaluation Study Group –

PRAISE. Effect of amlodipine on morbidity and mortality in severe chronic heart failure. *N Engl J Med* 1996; **335:** 1107–14.

8. Hampton JR, van Veldhuisen DJ, Kleber FX. Randomised study of effect of ibopamine on survival in patients with advanced severe heart failure. *Lancet* 1997; 349: 971–7.

9. Cohn JN, Goldstein SO, Greenberg BH, et al. A dose-dependent increase in mortality with vesnarinone among patients with severe heart failure. *N Engl J Med* 1998; **339:** 1810–16.

10. Yusuf S. Effect of enalapril on survival in patients with reduced left ventricular ejection fractions and congestive heart failure. *N Engl J Med* 1991; **325:** 293–302.

11. Hjalmarson A, Goldstein S, Fagerberg B, et al. Effects of controlled-release metoprolol on total mortality, hospitalizations, and well-being in patients with heart failure: the Metoprolol CR/XL Randomized Intervention Trial in congestive heart failure (MERIT-HF). MERIT-HF Study Group. *JAMA* 2000; **283:** 1295–302.

12. Perry G, Brown E, Thornton R, et al. The effect of digoxin on mortality and morbidity in patients with heart failure. *N Engl J Med* 1997; **336:** 525–33.

13. Erdmann E, Lechat P, Verkenne P, Wiemann H. Results from posthoc analyses of the CIBIS II trial: effect of bisoprolol in high-risk patient groups with chronic heart failure. *Eur J Heart Fail* 2001; **3:** 469–79.

14. Lechat P, Hulot JS, Escolano S, et al. Heart rate and cardiac rhythm relationships with bisoprolol benefit in chronic heart failure in CIBIS II Trial. *Circulation* 2001; **103:** 1428–33.

15. Reduced costs with bisoprolol treatment for heart failure: an economic analysis of the second Cardiac Insufficiency Bisoprolol Study (CIBIS-II). *Eur Heart J* 2001; **22:** 1021–31.

Metoprolol

Metoprolol has been licensed for the treatment of hypertension in some countries since 1975. It is a lipophilic, beta$_1$ selective adrenoceptor blocking drug with a short half-life. For many years, long acting preparations have been available but more recently a true controlled release preparation metoprolol CR/XL has been developed. This provides low even plasma concentrations over 24 hours[1] and was the preparation used in the MERIT-HF trial.[2] In earlier studies, metoprolol has been shown to reduce coronary mortality and sudden death in hypertensive patients,[3,4] and post-MI patients,[5,6] and to reduce the combined endpoint of death and need for cardiac transplantation in patients with heart failure.[7]

MERIT-HF

The primary objective of MERIT-HF was to examine the effect of metoprolol, added to conventional therapy, on all-cause mortality in patients with moderately severe symptomatic chronic heart failure caused by reduced left ventricular systolic function. It was a large randomized, multicentre (313 sites in 12 European countries and the USA) and details of the trial are presented in Appendix Tables A1–A7.

A total of 3991 patients were enrolled; the inclusion criteria are set out in Appendix Table A2. All patients had an ejection fraction of 0.4 or less, they were in a stable clinical condition and metoprolol CR/XL was started at a dose of 12.5 mg daily (or 25 mg for NYHA Class II patients). The dose was increased slowly to a target dose of 200 mg daily.

Results

The study was stopped prematurely on the recommendation of the independent safety committee. 3980 patient years had been accumulated and the mean follow-up time was 1 year. The trial profile is shown in Figure 22. The cumulative mortality curves are presented in Figure 23. A total of 145 patients on metoprolol and 217 patients on placebo died ($p = 0.00009$, $p = 0.0062$ after adjustment for interim analysis). The mortality rates were 7.2% and 11% per patient year of follow-up with a relative risk of 0.66 (95% CI 0.53–0.81). There were fewer sudden deaths in

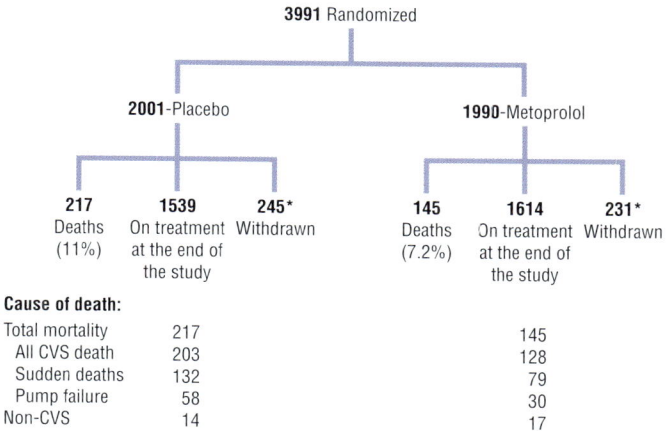

Figure 22
MERIT-HF trial profile.

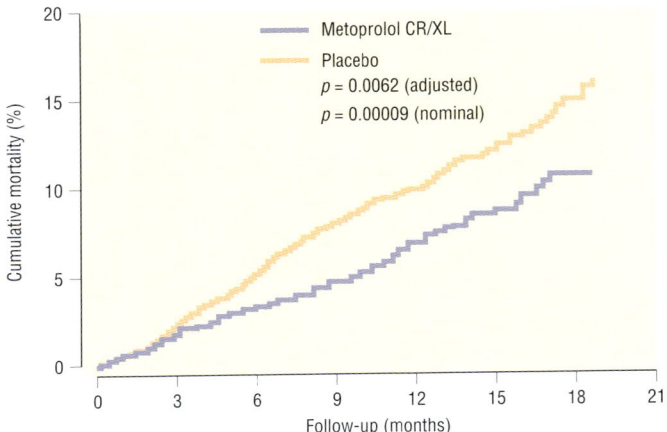

Figure 23
Cumulative mortality curves in MERIT-HF. p values adjusted for two interim analyses.

the metoprolol group, 79 versus 132 (RR = 0.59, 95% CI 0.45–0.78, $p < 0.0002$). Deaths from aggravated heart failure were 30 on metoprolol and 58 on placebo with a relative risk of 0.51 (95% CI 0.33–0.79, $p = 0.0023$).

The numbers of hospital admissions for worsening heart failure were 317 on metoprolol and 451 on placebo, the number of days in hospital being 3401 and 5303.

Detailed evaluation of the MERIT-HF trial

In this section the design and results of MERIT-HF[2] are compared with the US carvedilol Programme (USCP),[8] the bisoprolol trial (CIBIS-II)[9] and the COPERNICUS trials. The details of the design, conduct and inclusion criteria of the four trials are presented in Appendix Tables A1 and A2. The characteristics of the patients enrolled, endpoints and annual mortality rates are set out in Appendix Table A3 and the concomitant medication in Appendix Table A4.

Entry criteria

The enrolment criteria were very similar to those in CIBIS-II and the USCP (Appendix Tables A1 and A2).[8,9] There were only three notable differences. Patients with higher LVEF (≤0.40 versus 0.35) could be enrolled in MERIT-HF, but only if they had a reduced exercise capacity. While CIBIS-II recruited NYHA Class III and IV patients, MERIT-HF could recruit NYHA Class II–IV patients. Patients in MERIT-HF were also required to have a higher resting heart rate than those in CIBIS-II (≥68 versus ≥60 beats/minute). Patients were enrolled after a 2-week single-blind placebo period. The enrollment criteria for MERIT-HF differed considerably from COPERNICUS. COPERNICUS required patients to have more severe CHF, a lower LVEF (<0.25) and allowed randomizations of patients with a lower systolic blood pressure (≥ 85 mmHg compared to ≥ 100 mmHg).

Details of patients

MERIT-HF recruited the most patients of the four trials (3991 patients were randomized from 8192 screened). The average age of patients was higher than in the other trials and MERIT-HF recruited a smaller proportion of NYHA Class III patients (and a greater proportion of Class II patients), by design, than CIBIS-II (Appendix Tables A2–A4). Blood pressure, heart rate and LVEF were similar to CIBIS-II, as was concomitant medical therapy. In keeping with the different entry criteria, the patients enrolled in COPERNICUS had a much lower mean LVEF than in MERIT-HF (0.20 versus 0.28) though surprisingly had a higher mean systolic blood pressure than the patients in MERIT-HF (123 versus 117 mmHg).

Event rates

In keeping with the broader enrolment criteria in MERIT-HF (class II–IV versus III–IV and higher LVEF) annual mortality was a little lower than in CIBIS-II (11.0% versus 13.2%, Appendix Table A3).[2,9] In the placebo group, the mortality rate in NYHA Class II, III and IV patients was 7.1%, 13.2% and 24.9% per patient year of follow-up, respectively. The rates in Class III and IV patients in CIBIS-II were very similar at 15.8% and 24.6%. COPERNICUS patients, all of whom had symptomatic limitation equivalent to NYHA Class III and IV, had an annual mortality rate of 18.5% in the placebo group. The proportion of patients dying suddenly in MERIT-HF was greater than in CIBIS-II (61% versus 36% in the respective placebo groups), in keeping with the higher proportion of NYHA Class II patients. Patients with milder heart failure are more likely to die suddenly whereas those with more severe heart failure are more likely to die from progressive pump failure (Appendix Table A5).[2,9]

Follow-up

Average follow-up in MERIT-HF was slightly shorter than in CIBIS-II (1.0 versus 1.3 years)[2,9] and slightly longer than in COPERNICUS (about 10.4 months). No patients were lost to follow-up.

Haemodynamic effects

After 6 months, heart rate fell by 3 beats/minute in the placebo group compared with 14 beats/minute in the metoprolol group ($p < 0.0001$).[2] This was very similar to the changes in heart rate in the USCP (a reduction of 1.4 and 12.6 beats/minute in the placebo and carvedilol groups respectively; $p < 0.001$).[8] Remarkably, there was a smaller reduction in systolic blood pressure in the metoprolol group (–2.1 mmHg) than in the placebo group (–3.5 mmHg; $p = 0.013$). Blood pressure did not change significantly in either treatment group in the USCP.[8]

Effects on mortality

Metoprolol reduced total mortality by 34% (relative risk 0.66, 95% CI 0.53-0.81), a treatment effect identical to that of bisoprolol in CIBIS-II and carvedilol in COPERNICUS (Figure 23).[2,9] Metoprolol also had a broadly similar effect to bisoprolol on specific causes and modes of death (Appendix Table A5). In particular, the risk of sudden death was substantially reduced. The mortality benefit was seen across a wide range of patient sub-groups (Figure 24).[2] An interesting new, post hoc, analysis of the effect of metoprolol in the most severely ill MERIT-HF patients, including 'COPERNICUS-like' patients has been published recently. This showed that metoprolol reduces mortality (and morbidity) regardless of baseline heart failure severity.[10]

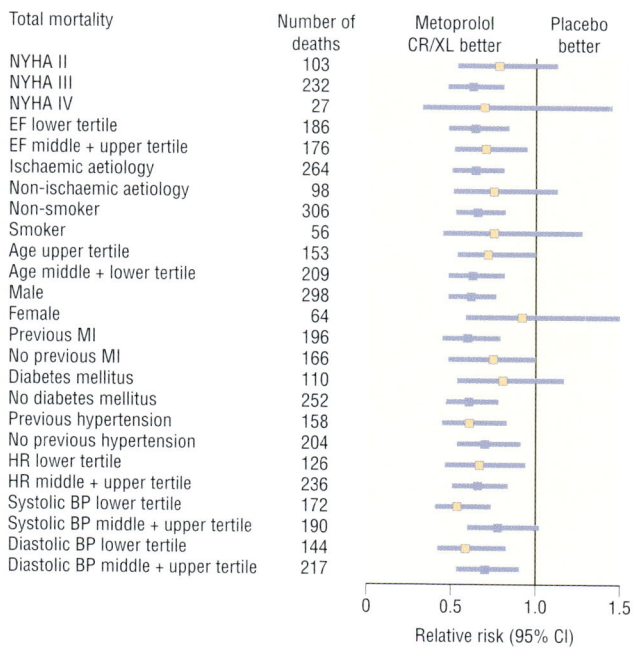

Figure 24
MERIT-HF: total mortality in subgroups.

Effects on morbidity

Hospital admission and other morbidities were not reported in the principal MERIT-HF results paper but have been published subsequently (Figures 25–27).[11] Both cardiovascular hospital admissions and hospital admissions for worsening heart failure were significantly reduced by metoprolol (Figure 25). These findings are similar to those in the USCP (30% reduction in cardiovascular hospital admissions and a 53% (95% CI 19–70) reduction in CHF hospital admissions). The combined endpoint of any death or hospital admission for any cause was also reduced by 19% with metoprolol (Figure 26, $p = 0.00012$).

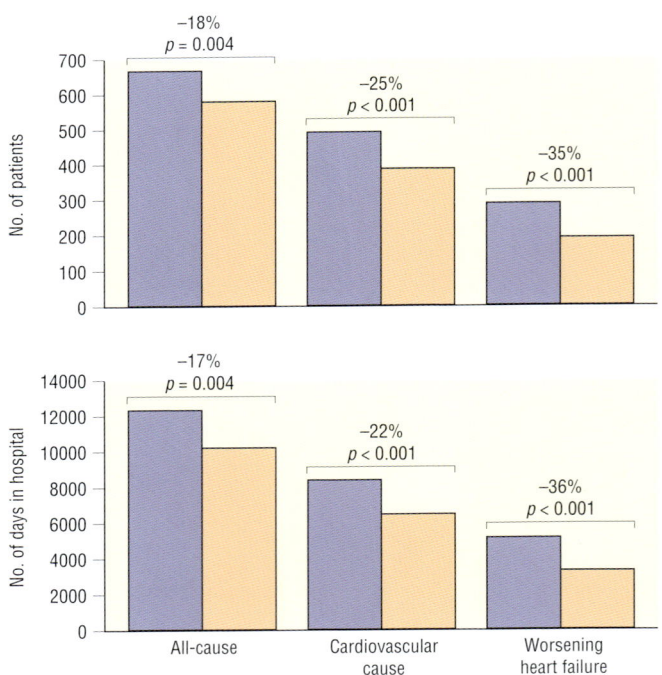

Figure 25
MERIT-HF: number of patients admitted to hospital and total number of days spent in the hospital due to any cause, cardiovascular causes or worsening heart failure. Intervention: ■, placebo; ■, metoprolol CR/XL.

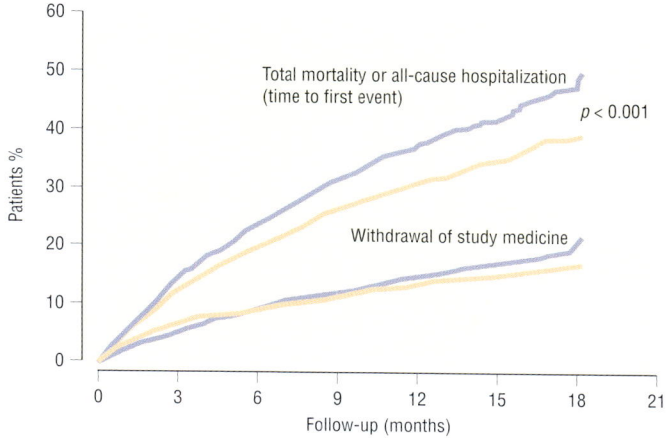

Figure 26
Cumulative percentages (time to first event) for the combined endpoint of total mortality or all-cause hospitalization and cumulative withdrawals from studying medication in MERIT-HF. Intervention: —, placebo; —, metoprolol CR/XL.

Effects on functional class, quality of life and exercise tolerance

Though not reported in the main MERIT-HF report, the subsequent publication on morbidity also shows that metoprolol also improved NYHA functional class ($p = 0.0028$) and quality of life (Figure 27, $p = 0.0089$) as measured using the McMaster Overall Treatment Evaluation questionnaire (OTE).[10] The OTE was used in a sub-group of 741 patients. Of the 185 metoprolol CR/XL treated patients who reported an improvement in quality of life, 71% judged this improvement as important or extremely important for carrying out daily activities.

A peak oxygen consumption sub-study of MERIT-HF has recently been published, showing no effect of metoprolol over placebo.[12]

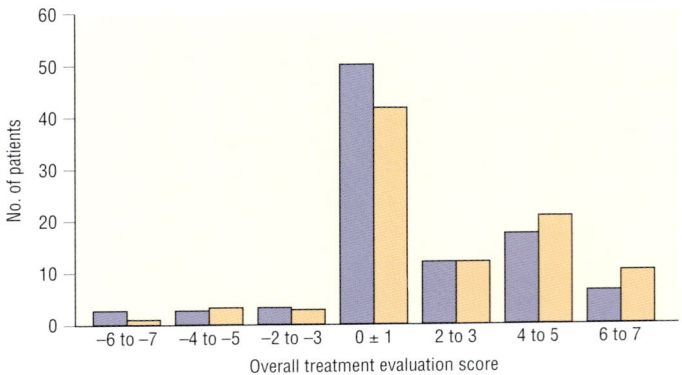

Figure 27
Overall treatment evaluation score as judged by patients at the end of the study.
Intervention: ■, placebo; ■, metoprolol CR/XL.

Dosing

The target dose of slow release metoprolol in MERIT-HF was 200 mg od.[2] The mean dose achieved in the active therapy group was 159 mg compared with 179 mg in the placebo group (Appendix Table A6). 64% of metoprolol-treated patients and 82% of placebo-treated patients reached the target dose. 91% of the placebo group and 87% of the metoprolol group were titrated to a maintenance dose of 100 mg or more (half the target dose). The proportion of patients reaching higher maintenance doses was greater than in CIBIS-II but smaller than in the USCP (Appendix Table A6).[2,8,9] The design of the USCP, with an open-label run-in period, will, however, almost certainly have inflated the proportion reaching target in the carvedilol studies.

In COPERNICUS, 65.1% of patients were titrated, at some stage in the first 4 months of the trial, to the target carvedilol dose of 25mg bd (the equivalent figure for placebo was 78.2%).

Tolerability and adverse effects

The principal MERIT-HF results paper reports that study drug was permanently discontinued, early, in 15.3% of the placebo group and 13.9% of the metoprolol group (0.90, 95% CI 0.77–1.06). This is very similar to the proportion of patients stopping treatment prematurely in CIBIS-II (15% in both treatment groups). Adverse effects are not reported in the principal MERIT-HF results paper but are detailed in the subsequent morbidity analysis (Table A7).[10] Permanent withdrawal of study drug for any adverse event occurred in 196 (9.8%) patients in the placebo group and 234 (11.7%) patients in the metoprolol CR/XL group. These rates are very similar to those seen in the shorter duration USCP (7.8% placebo and 5.7% carvedilol) though it must be remembered that the USCP open-label run-in phase will have selected patients able to tolerate carvedilol. In COPERNICUS, 14.8% of carvedilol-treated and 18.5% of placebo-treated patients had been withdrawn from randomized therapy. *Overall rates* of specific adverse effects are not given for MERIT-HF to compare with the USCP and CIBIS-II. The most frequent specific adverse reactions *leading to treatment discontinuation* are, however, reported. It is clear that adverse events severe enough to lead to treatment discontinuation were infrequent in both USCP and MERIT-HF. Heart failure was less frequent on active therapy in both trials (3.9% of metoprolol CR/XL and 5.8% of placebo-treated patients; 2.3% placebo and 1.6% of carvedilol-treated patients in USCP; data not available for CIBIS-II). There was a small excess of bradycardia and dizziness in both studies though, interestingly, neither dizziness nor hypotension seemed to be more common with carvedilol, despite its alpha adrenoceptor blocking activity, though, again, the possible bias caused by the open-label run-in phase of the USCP must be taken into account.

References

1. Kendall MJ. Metoprolol CR/ZOK – its role and efficacy: a review article. *J Clin Pharmacol* 1990; **30**: S57–S60.
2. MERIT-HF Study Group. Effect of metoprolol CR/XL in chronic heart failure: metoprolol CR/XL randomised intervention trial in congestive heart failure (MERIT-HF). *Lancet* 1999; **353**: 2001–7.
3. Wikstrand J, Warnold I, Olsson G, Toumilehto J, Elmfeldt D, Berglund G. Primary prevention with metoprolol in patients with hypertension. Mortality results from the MAPHY study. *JAMA* 1988; **259**: 1976–82.
4. Olsson G, Tuomilehto J, Berglund G, et al. Primary prevention of sudden cardiovascular death in hypertensive patients: mortality results from the MAPHY study. *Am J Hypert* 1991; **4**: 151–8.
5. Olsson G, Wikstrand J, Warnold I, et al. Metoprolol-induced reduction in postinfarction mortality: pooled results from five double-blind randomized trials. *Eur Heart J* 1992; **13**: 28–32.
6. Kendall MJ, Lynch KP, Hjalmarson A, Kjekshus J. Beta-blockers and sudden cardiac death. *Ann Intern Med* 1995; **123**: 358–67.
7. Waagstein F, Bristow M, Swedberg K, et al, and the Metoprolol Dilated Cardiomyopathy (MDC) trial study group. Beneficial effects of metoprolol in idiopathic dilated cardiomyopathy. *Lancet* 1993; **342**: 1441–6.
8. Packer M, Bristow MR, Cohn JN, et al, and the US Carvedilol Heart Failure Study Group. The effect of carvedilol on morbidity and mortality in patients with chronic heart failure. *N Engl J Med* 1996; **334**: 1349–55.
9. CIBIS-II Investigators and Committees. The cardiac insufficiency bisoprolol study II (CIBIS-II): a randomised trial. *Lancet* 1999; **353**: 9–13.
10. Goldstein S, Fagerberg B, Hjalmarson A, et al. Metoprolol controlled release/extended release in patients with severe heart failure. Analysis of the experience in the MERIT-HF study. *J Am Coll Cardiol* 2001; **38**: 932–8.
11. Hjalmarson A, Goldstein S, Fagerberg B, et al. Effects of controlled-release metoprolol on total mortality, hospitalizations, and well-being in patients with heart failure: the Metoprolol CR/XL Randomized Intervention Trial in congestive heart failure (MERIT-HF). MERIT-HF Study Group. *JAMA* 2000; **283**: 1295–302.
12. Gullestad L, Manhenke C, Aarsland T, et al. Effect of metoprolol CR/XL on exercise tolerance in chronic heart failure - a substudy to the MERIT-HF trial. *Eur J Heart Fail* 2001; **3**: 463–8.

What we still don't know about beta-blockers in CHF

All four main trials recruited relatively young patients, though sub-group analyses of MERIT-HF, the USCP, and COPERNICUS suggest that benefit is obtained in both younger and older patients.[1–3]

Similarly, all four trials recruited few female patients (about 20% in total). Because of this there is some uncertainty about the benefit in women. The USCP suggests a greater benefit in women than men (though the numbers are extremely small).[1] MERIT-HF showed a trend in the opposite direction.[2] The main CIBIS-II report does not give a breakdown of results by sex, but a subsequent report has suggested women get a greater benefit from bisoprolol than men.[3] Similarly, there is uncertainty about some important sub-sets of patients, e.g., those with atrial fibrillation. Formal meta-analysis should shed more light on these issues. We also do not know about more rapid treatment titration schedules.

To date, there is no good evidence to show that any of the beta-blockers used in the four main trials are more efficacious or better tolerated than one another, though the COMET trial to compare short-acting metoprolol with-carvedilol may shed some light on this.

Conclusions

It seems quite clear from the data presented that beta-blockers substantially reduce mortality and morbidity in patients with stable NYHA Class II and III CHF due to left ventricular systolic dysfunction of all causes (Table 12).[1–3] These large trials are supported by meta-analyses of smaller studies.[4,5] The mortality benefit is probably a little larger than that obtained with ACE inhibitors. The mortality benefit in patients with severe CHF is even greater. Treatment of 1000 COPERNICUS-like patients for 1 year prevented

Table 12
Events prevented per 1000 patients years of treatment

	ACE-I (1)	Beta-blockers (2)	(3)	Spironolactone (4)	Digoxin (5)
Hospital admissions (any cause)	99	65	N/A	138	40
Deaths	13	38	71	57	0

(1) based on the treatment arm of the SOLVD – average follow-up 3.5 years
(2) based on the MERIT-HF study – average follow-up 1 year
(3) based on COPERNICUS trial, using annualized rates – average follow-up 10.4 months
(4) based on the RALES trial – average follow-up 2 years
(5) based on the DIG trial – average follow-up 3 years.
Note: (a) shorter follow-up tends to exaggerate benefit; (b) absolute benefit is a function of absolute risk — RALES and COPERNICUS recruited much higher risk patients (NYHA Class III/IV) than the other trials (mainly NYHA Class II/III; (c) digoxin, beta-blockers and spironolactone have largely been evaluated in addition to ACE inhibitors. N/A = not available.

Table 13

*Initiating dose, target dose, and titration scheme of beta-blocking agents in placebo controlled large trials**

β-blocker	First dose (mg)	Titration scheme daily dose (mg) [†]									Target total daily dose (mg)
		Wk1	Wk2	Wk3	Wk4	Wk5	Wk6	Wk7	Wk8–11	Wk 12–15	
Metoprolol (MERIT-HF)	25[‡]	25	25	50	50	100	100	200			200
Bisoprolol (CIBIS-II)	1.25	1.25	2.5	3.75	5.0				7.5	10	10
COPERNICUS	3.125	3.125	3.125	6.25	6.25	12.5	12.5	25	25		50[¶]

*Forced titration in all studies, assuming preceding dose tolerated.
[†]Dose once daily for metoprolol and bisoprolol and twice daily for carvedilol.
[‡]Slow release (metoprolol CR/XL) formulation 12.5 mg recommended in NYHA class III–IV patients.
[¶]In two doses: 25 mg bid except for patients >85 kg where the dose may be increased to 50 mg bid.

70 premature deaths. This compares to 57 premature deaths avoided per 1000 patient years of treatment in RALES.

On the whole, initiated at a low dose and titrated slowly, beta-blockers are well tolerated in CHF, though perhaps a little less well than ACE inhibitors. All the evidence shows that all stable NYHA Class II–III CHF patients with reduced left ventricular systolic function should receive a beta-blocker, in addition to standard therapy (including an ACE inhibitor), unless there is a specific contraindication (eg, asthma). Treatment should be used according to the dosing regimen and titration protocol used in one of the three large mortality studies (Table 13). Although there may still be some debate about initiating treatment in unstable patients with more severe symptoms, the clear message of the recent trials is that patients should be started on a beta-blocker as early as possible in the course of their disease so that such a debate never arises.

References

1. Packer M, Bristow MR, Cohn JN, et al, and the US Carvedilol Heart Failure Study Group. The effect of carvedilol on morbidity and mortality in patients with chronic heart failure. *N Engl J Med* 1996; **334:** 1349–55.
2. MERIT-HF Study Group. Effect of metoprolol CR/XL in chronic heart failure: metoprolol CR/XL randomised intervention trial in congestive heart failure (MERIT-HF). *Lancet* 1999; **353:** 2001–7.
3. Simon T, Mary-Krause M, Funck-Brentano C, Jaillon P. Sex differences in the prognosis of congestive heart failure. Results from the Cardiac Insufficiency Bisoprolol Study (CIBIS-II). *Circulation* 2001; **103:** 375.
4. Cohn JN. Safety and efficacy of carvedilol in severe heart failure. The US Carvedilol Heart Failure Study Group. *J Cardiol Fail* 1997; **3**(3): 173–9.
5. The CIBIS II Scientific Committee. Design of the Cardiac Insufficiency Bisoprolol Study II (CIBIS II). *Fund Clin Pharmacol* 1997; **11**(2):138–42.

Trial acronyms used

ELITE	Evaluation of Losartan in the Elderly
PROMISE	Prospective Randomized Milrinone Survival Evaluation
PRAISE	Prospective Randomized Amlodipine Survival Evaluation
PRIME	Prospective Randomized study of Ibopamine on Mortality and Efficacy
DIG	Digitalis Investigation Group
PRECISE	Prospective Randomized Evaluation of Carvedilol on Symptoms and Exercise
BEST	Beta-blocker Evaluation Survival Trial
RALES	Randomized Aldactone Evaluation Study

Appendix A

BEST

One other large beta-blocker trial did not show a reduction in all cause mortality with bucindolol, a non-selective, vasodilating beta-blocker. Cardiovascular events were, however, reduced and the findings of BEST[1] were broadly in keeping with other studies reviewed. Why BEST showed no mortality benefit is uncertain. Whether this reflected the drug used or the patients enrolled (there were more African Americans than in the other studies and these patients may not have had a benefit from beta-blocker) has been debated a lot. Bucindolol is not being developed further for CHF.

Reference

1. A trial of the beta-blocker bucindolol in patients with advanced chronic heart failure. *N Engl J Med* 2001; **344**:1659–67.

Table A1
Design and conduct of beta-blocker heart failure trials

	USCP	CIBIS-II	MERIT-HF	COPERNICUS	BEST
Estimated annual mortality in placebo group (%)	12.0	11.2	9.4	28	15
Estimated risk reduction with beta-blocker (%)	n/a*	25	30	20	25
Estimated duration of trial (years)					
Recruitment	---	1	1.2	2.75	4.5
Follow-up	---	2	2.5	1.5	3.0
					3.0
Estimated number of patients required	1101	2500	3500	2500	2800
Power of study to detect pre-specified risk reduction (%)	n/a†	95	80	90	85
Early stopping rules for benefit (significance level)	No	Yes (p < 0.001)	Yes (p < 0.0036)	Yes	Yes
Recruitment started	23 April, 93	27 November, 95	14 February, 97	28 October, 97	30 May, 95
Recruitment stopped	n/a††	13 May, 97	14 April, 98	20 March, 00	31 Dec, 98
Study programme stopped prematurely	Yes	Yes	Yes	Yes	Yes
Date study stopped	3 February, 95	5 March, 98	31 October, 98	20 March, 00	29 July, 99

*Trial designed to exclude a 33% increase in mortality; † 95% power to detect a 33% increase in mortality; †† some component studies still recruiting at time USCP terminated.
--- Data not available.

Table A2
*Inclusion criteria for beta-blockers heart failure trials**

	USCP	CIBIS-II	MERIT-HF	COPERNICUS	BEST
Age (years)	18–85	18–80	40–80	≥18	≥18
NYHA class	II–IV	III–IV	II–IV	III–IV[††††]	II–IV
Duration of CHF (months)	3	3	3	3	Not required
Stability (weeks)	4	2	2	1	4
Diuretic	Required	Required	Required	Required	Optional
ACE inhibitor	Required	Required	Required	Required	Required
Digoxin	Optional	Optional	Optional	Optional	Required[†]
Calcium antagonists	None	None	Rate limiting excluded	None	None
Antiarrhythmic drugs	Classic Ic & III excluded[††]	Amiodarone only	No amiodarone within 6 months	Amiodarone only	None

*All enrolled men and women; [†]2% in both treatment groups received dihydropyridines; [††]class III includes amiodarone; **50 mg b.i.d for patients ≥ 85 kg; ***Slow release formulation of metoprolol CR/XL; [+]Until November, 1996 (92% received); [+++]100 mg b.i.d. if > 75 kg. [††††]"symptoms of dyspnoea and/or fatigue at rest or on minimal exertion for at least 2 months".
--- Data not yet available.

Table A2
Continued

	USCP	CIBIS-II	MERIT-HF	COPERNICUS	BEST
LVEF	≤0.35	≤ 0.35	≤0.40	<0.25	≤ 0.35
6 minute walk	All (various criteria)	Not required	<450 m if LVEF 0.360–0.40	Not required	Not required
Heart rate (beats/min)	68	≥60	≥68	≥68	50
Systolic blood pressure (mm Hg)	≥ 85	≥100	≥100	≥85	≥80
Tolerability of beta-blocker (open-label run-in)	Required	Not required	Not required	Not required	Not required
Target dose (mg)	25/50mg bid**	10 mg od	200 mg od ***	25 mg bid	+++ 50/100 mg bid

*All enrolled men and women; †2% in both treatment groups received dihydropyridines; ††class III includes amiodarone; **50 mg b.i.d for patients ≥ 85 kg; ***Slow release formulation of metoprolol CR/XL; ⁺Until November, 1996 (92% received); +++100 mg b.i.d. if > 75 kg. ††††"symptoms of dyspnoea and/or fatigue at rest or on minimal exertion for at least 2 months".
--- Data not yet available.

Table A3
Characteristics of patients enrolled, endpoints, and annual mortality rates in the large beta-blocker trials in CHF

	USCP	CIBIS-II	MERIT-HF	COPERNICUS	BEST
Number of patients	1094	2647	3991	2289	2708
Mean age (years)	58	61	64	63	60
Male sex (%)	77	81	78	80	78
Mean LVEF (%)	23	28	28	20	23
Ischaemic heart disease	47	50 *	65	67	58
NYHA class (%)					
II	53	0	41	+++	0
III	44	83	56	+++	92
IV	3	17	3.6	+++	8
Mean systolic BP (mm Hg)	115	130	130	123	117
Mean diastolic BP (mm Hg)	73	80	78	76	71

*Strict criteria were used to diagnose ischaemic heart disease in CIBIS-II; **Estimated annual mortality rate in CIBIS-II and mortality rate per patient year in MERIT-HF; +Median follow up only 6.5 months; ++Median in case of USCP and COPERNICUS; +++"Symptoms of dyspnoea and/or fatigue at rest or on minimal exertion for at least 2 months". --- Data not yet available.

Table A3
Continued

	USCP	CIBIS-II	MERIT-HF	COPERNICUS	BEST
Mean heart rate (beats/min)	83	81	82	80	82
Atrial fibrillation	---	20	17	---	12
Diabetes mellitus	---	---	25	---	36
Hypertension	---	---	44	---	---
Primary endpoint	Various	Mortality	Mortality	Mortality	Mortality
Total number of deaths	54	384	362	320	856
Annual mortality rate **					
Placebo	n/a [+]	13.2	11.0	18.5	16.6
Beta-blocker	n/a [+]	8.8	7.2	11.4	14.9
Mean follow-up	6.5 months	1.3 years	1 year	10.4 months	2 years

*Strict criteria were used to diagnose ischaemic heart disease in CIBIS-II; **Estimated annual mortality rate in CIBIS-II and mortality rate per patient year in MERIT-HF; [+]Median follow up only 6.5 months; [++]Median in case of USCP and COPERNICUS; [+++]"Symptoms of dyspnoea and/or fatigue at rest or on minimal exertion for at least 2 months".
--- Data not yet available.

Table A4

Beta-blocker heart failure trials: concomitant medication

	USCP	CIBIS-II*	MERIT-HF	COPERNICUS	BEST
Diuretic	95**	99	91	99	94
ACE inhibitor	95	96	90[+]	97[†††]	91
Digoxin	91	52	64	66	92
Aspirin/antiplatelet agents	---	41[††]	46	---	45
Nitrates/direct acting vasodilators	32[†]	58	---	20	47
Spironolactone	---	10	7	20	4

* CIBIS-II permitted amiodarone (which the other two trials did not) – 15% received this drug; ** Loop diuretic; [+]96 % ACE inhibitor or angiotensin II receptor antagonist; [†††]ACE inhibitor or angiotensin II receptor antagonist; [††]Antiplatelet agents in CIBIS-II; [†]Direct acting vasodilators in USCP.
--- Data not yet available.

Table A5
Analysis of mortality data in three large beta-blocker trials

	USCP		CIBIS-II		MERIT-HF		COPERNICUS		BEST	
	Placebo (n=398)	Carvedilol (n=696)	Placebo (n=1320)	Bisoprolol (n=1327)	Placebo (n=2001)	Metoprolol (n=1990)	Placebo (n=1133)	Carvedilol (n=1156)	Placebo (n=1354)	Bucindolol (n=1354)
All	31	22	228	156	217	145	--	--	449	411
Cardiovascular (%)*	31 (100)	20 (91)	161 (71)	119 (76)	203 (94)	128 (88)	--	--	389 (87)	342 (83)
Sudden death (%)†	15 (48)	12 (55)	83 (36)	48 (31)	132 (61)	79 (54)	--	--	203 (45)	182 (44)
Pump failure (%)**††	13 (42)	5 (23)	47 (21)	36 (23)	58 (27)	30 (21)	--	--	140 (31)	122 (30)

*CIBIS-II hazard ratio 0.71, 95% CI 0.56 to 0.90, p=0.0049; MERIT-HF relative risk 0.62, 95% CI 0.50 to 0.78, p = 0.0003.
†CIBIS-II hazard ratio 0.56, 95% CI 0.39 to 0.80, p=0.0011; MERIT-HF relative risk 0.45, 95% CI 0.45 to 0.78, p = 0.0002.
††CIBIS-II hazard ratio 0.74, 95% CI 0.48 to 1.14, p=0.17; MERIT-HF relative risk 0.51, 95% CI 0.33 to 0.79, p = 0.0023.
**Pump failure equates to progressive or worsening heart failure.
-- Data not yet available.
NA, not available

Table A6
Treatment dosing in the large beta-blocker mortality trials

	USCP	CIBIS-II	MERIT-HF	COPERNICUS*
Proportion of patients reaching target dose in beta-blocker group (%)	80	43	64	65.1
Proportion of patients reaching half or more of target dose (%)	---	67	87	---
Mean dose in beta-blocker group (mg)	45	---	159	37
Proportion stopping treatment early (%)				
Placebo	18	15	15.3	18.5
Beta-blocker	11	15	13.9	14.8

*Proportion reaching dose at some point in the first 4 months of trial, proportion withdrawing at one year.
--- Data not yet available.

Table A7
Adverse event rates (%)

	USCP*		CIBIS-II†		MERIT-HF††		COPERNICUS	
	Placebo	Carvedilol	Placebo	Bisoprolol	Placebo	Metoprolol	Placebo	Carvedilol
Heart failure	21 (2.3)	16 (1.6)	23	18	5.8	3.9	---	---
Dyspnoea	25 (1.0)	22 (0.3)	17	14	0.6	0.8	---	---
Dizziness	20 (0)	33 (0.4)	10	13	0.3	0.6	---	---
Bradycardia	1 (0)	9 (0.9)	5	15	0.2	0.8	---	---
Hypotension	4 (0.3)	9 (0.3)	7	11	0.2	0.6	---	---
Fatigue	23 (0.8)	25 (0.7)	7	9	0.4	0.7	---	---

Data are number of patients. *Most frequent adverse reactions. ( ) = leading to discontinuation of double blind treatment; †most frequent adverse reactions; †† most frequent adverse reactions leading to withdrawal of study drug. --- Data not yet available.

Appendix B

References

1. McMurray J, Cohen-Solal A, Dietz R, et al. Practical recommendations for the use of ACE inhibitors, beta-blockers and spironolactone in heart failure: putting guidelines into practice. *Eur J Heart Fail* 2000; **3:** 495–502.
2. A trial of the beta-blocker bucindolol in patients with advanced chronic heart failure. *N Engl J Med* 2001; **344:** 1659–67.
3. Dargie HJ. Effect of carvedilol on outcome after myocardial infarction in patients with left-ventricular dysfunction the CAPRICORN randomised trial. *Lancet* 2001; **357:** 1385–90.

Table B1

Practical guidance on the use of beta-blockers in patients with CHF due to left ventricular systolic dysfunction. Reproduced with permission from McMurray et al.[1]

Why?

Several major randomized controlled trials (i.e. USCP, CIBIS II, MERIT-HF, COPERNICUS) have shown, conclusively, that beta-blockers increase survival, reduce hospital admissions and improve NHYA class and quality of life when added to standard therapy (diuretics, digoxin and ACE inhibitors) in patients with stable mild and moderate CHF and in some patients with severe CHF. One other trial (BEST)[2] did not show a reduction in all cause mortality but did report a reduction in cardiovascular mortality and is other wise broadly consistent with the aforementioned studies. The recent CAPRICORN Study showed a reduction in mortality with carvedilol in post-myocardial infarction patients with reduced left ventricular systolic dysfunction.[3]

In whom and when?

Indications:	Potentially all patients with stable mild and moderate CHF; patients with severe CHF should be referred for specialist advice
	1st line treatment (along with ACE inhibitors) in patients with stable NYHA class I-IV CHF, start early as possible in course of disease
Contraindications:	Asthma
Cautions / seek specialist advice:	Severe (NYHA class IV) CHF
	Current or recent (< 4 weeks) exacerbation of CHF e.g. hospital admission with worsening CHF
	Heart block or heart rate < 60/min
	Persisting signs of congestion: raised jugular venous pressure, ascites, marked peripheral oedema
Drug interations to look out for:	Verapamil/diltiazem (should be discontinued)
	Amiodarone

Table B1
continued

Where?

In the community in stable patients (NYHA class IV/severe CHF patients should be referred for specialist advice)

Not in unstable patients hospitalized with worsening CHF

Other exceptions: see CAUTIONS/SEEK SPECIALIST ADVICE

Which beta-blocker and what dose?

Only three beta-blockers have been shown to reduce mortality in heart failure. There is evidence that some beta-blockers may be ineffective. The benefits of beta-blockers cannot be assumed to a class effect in heart failure

	Starting dose (mg)	Target dose (mg)
Bisoprolol	1.25 once daily	10 once daily
Carvedilol	3.125 twice daily	25–50 twice daily
Metoprolol CR/XL	12.5–25 once daily	200 once daily

How to use?

Start with a low dose (see above)

Double dose at not less than 2 weekly intervals

Aim for target dose (see above) or, failing that, the highest tolerated dose

Remember some beta-blocker is better than no beta-blocker

Table B1
continued

Monitor HR, BP, clinical status (symptoms, signs, especially signs of congestion, body weight)

Check blood chemistry 1–2 weeks after initiation and 1–2 weeks after final dose titration

A specialist CHF nurse may assist with patient education, follow-up (in person/by telephone) and dose uptitration

When to down-titrate/stop up-titration, see PROBLEM SOLVING

Advice to patient

Explain expected benefits (see WHY?)

Emphasize that treatment given as much to prevent worsening of CHF as to improve symptoms, beta-blockers also increase survival

If symptomatic improvement occurs, this may develop slowly 3–6 months or longer

Temporary symptomatic deterioration may occur (estimated 20–30% of cases) during initiation/up-titration phase

Advise patient to report deterioration (see PROBLEM SOLVING) and that deterioration (tiredness, fatigue, breathlessness) can usually be easily managed by adjustment of other medication; patients should be advised not to stop beta-blocker therapy without consulting their physician

Patients should be encouraged to weigh themselves daily (after waking, before dressing, after voiding, before eating) and to increase their diuretic dose should their weight, persistently (> 2 days), by > 1.5–2.0 kg

Problem Solving

Worsening symptoms / signs (e.g. increasing dyspnoea, fatigue, oedema, weight gain):

If increasing congestion double dose of diuretic and/or halve dose of beta-blocker (if increasing diuretic does not work)

Table B1
continued

If marked fatigue (and/or bradycardia, see below) half dose of beta-blocker (rarely necessary)

Review patient in 1–2 weeks; if not improved seek specialist advice

If serious deterioration halve dose of beta-blocker or stop this treatment (rarely necessary); seek specialist advice

Low heart rate:

If < 50 beats/min and worsening symptoms – halve dose beta-blockers or, if severe deterioration, stop beta-blocker (rarely necessary)

Review need for other heart rate slowing drugs e.g. digoxin, amiodarone, diltiazem

Arrange ECG to exclude heart block

Seek specialist advice

Asymptomatic low blood pressure:

Does not usually require any change in therapy

Symptomatic hypotension:

If dizziness, light-headedness and/or confusion and a low blood pressure reconsider need for nitrates, calcium channel blockers and other vasodilators

If no signs/symptoms of congestion consider reducing diuretic dose

If these measures do not solve problem seek specialist advice

NB: beta-blockers should not be stopped suddenly unless absolutely necessary (there is a risk of a 'rebound' increase in myocardial ischaemia/infarction and arrhythmias); ideally specialist advice should be sought before treatment discontinuation

Index

Page numbers in *italic* text refer to figures or tables